Atlas of Diagnostic Endoscopy
Third Edition

Atlas of Diagnostic Endoscopy
Third Edition

Dr Mohammad Ibrarullah, FACS, MS, MCh

Senior Consultant, Department of Surgical Gastroenterology,
Apollo Hospitals, Bhubaneswar, India
Formerly, Professor and Head of Surgical Gastroenterology
SV Institute of Medical Sciences, Tirupati, India
Sri Ramachandra Medical College & Research Institute, Chennai &
Hitech Medical College and Hospital, Bhubaneswar, India

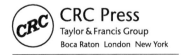

CRC Press
Taylor & Francis Group
Boca Raton London New York

CRC Press is an imprint of the
Taylor & Francis Group, an **informa** business

CRC Press
Taylor & Francis Group
6000 Broken Sound Parkway NW, Suite 300
Boca Raton, FL 33487-2742

First issued in paperback 2021

ISBN-13: 978-0-367-34500-6 (hbk)
ISBN-13: 978-1-03-208438-1 (pbk)

Library of Congress Cataloging-in-Publication Data

Names: Ibrarullah, Mohammad, author.
Title: Atlas of diagnostic endoscopy / by Dr. Mohammad Ibrarullah.
Description: 3 e. | Boca Raton : CRC Press, [2020] | Includes bibliographical references and index. |
Summary: "This book is a compilation of endoscopic images of the upper gastrointestinal tract.
The 3rd edition is enriched with high-resolution digital images highlighting the classification and staging of endoscopically relevant diseases. It outlines the technique and interpretation of such images proving to be a helpful guide to endoscopy practitioners"-- Provided by publisher.
Identifiers: LCCN 2019030549 (print) | LCCN 2019030550 (ebook) | ISBN 9780367345006
(hardback : alk. paper) | ISBN 9780429326240 (ebook)
Subjects: MESH: Gastrointestinal Diseases--diagnosis | Endoscopy, Gastrointestinal--methods |
Upper Gastrointestinal Tract--surgery | Atlas
Classification: LCC RC816 (print) | LCC RC816 (ebook) | NLM WI 17 | DDC 616.3/3--dc23
LC record available at https://lccn.loc.gov/2019030549
LC ebook record available at https://lccn.loc.gov/2019030550

Visit the Taylor & Francis Web site at
http://www.taylorandfrancis.com

and the CRC Press Web site at
http://www.crcpress.com

Contents

List of abbreviations

ACG	American College of Gastroenterology
AGA	American Gastroenterological Association
ASGE	American Society for Gastrointestinal Endoscopy
CMV	Cytomegalovirus
CT	Computed tomography
D1	1st part of duodenum
D2	2nd part of duodenum
EVL	Endoscopic variceal band ligation
FB	Foreign body
GAVE	Gastric antral vascular ectasia
GI	Gastrointestinal
GE	Gastroesophageal
GERD	Gastroesophageal reflux disease
GIST	Gastrointestinal stromal tumor
GJ	Gastrojejunostomy
GOV	Gastroesophageal varix
HIV	Human immunodeficiency virus
HPF	High-power field
HSV	Herpes simplex virus
IGV	Isolated gastric varix
LES	Lower esophageal sphincter
LPF	Left pyriform fossa
NET	Neuroendocrine tumor
NSAID	Nonsteroidal anti-inflammatory drug
PEG	Percutaneous endoscopic gastrostomy
PHG	Portal hypertensive gastropathy
RPF	Right pyriform fossa
TEF	Tracheoesophageal fistula
UGI	Upper gastrointestinal

Preface

Each passing year has seen tremendous advances in the field of both diagnostic and therapeutic endoscopy. While preparing the current edition of the atlas, I also felt tempted to add a few chapters on recent advances such as fluorescent endoscopy, magnification endoscopy, etc. However, on second thought I decided to restrict myself to basic endoscopy since my target readers, as I mentioned in the first edition of the atlas, are the "young doctors who wish to get initiated and practice endoscopy." The aim of this atlas is to provide them a strong foundation by familiarizing them with the basic concepts of endoscopy and aiding in correct interpretation of the pathology. Notwithstanding the number of similar atlases available online, it is always quick and easy to refer to a printed copy that is lying in the endoscopist's consultation chamber. Needless to say, printed images provide a longer-lasting impression as compared with those seen on the computer screen. Effort has been made to replace some poor quality and repetitive images of the previous edition with new ones, giving a fresh look to the current edition of the atlas. I sincerely hope that the atlas, in its current form, will find wide acceptance amongst endoscopy practitioners.

Acknowledgments

Those who provided professional, academic and technical support in compiling the atlas are

Prof. B Krishna Rau, Chennai
Prof. SR Naik, Lucknow
Dr D Srinivasa, Bangalore
Dr Gajanan Wagholikar, Pune
Dr Anuj Sarkari, Gorakhpur
Dr Amaresh Mishra, Bhubaneswar
Dr Anwar Basha, Tirupati
Dr T Shyamsundar, Nellore
Dr B Visweswara Rao, Srikakulum
Dr D Vijay Nagaraj, Cudappa
Dr D Gopikrishna Reddy, Tirupati
Dr M Srinivas, Rajmundry
TL Varalakshmi, Tirupati
V Dhanalakshmi, Tirupati
Dr Sidhant Kar, Bhubaneswar
Dr JM Rao, Bhubaneswar
Dr Neeraj K Mishra, Bhubaneswar
Dr Ambica P Das, Bhubaneswar
Dr Tapas Mishra, Bhubaneswar
Dr Sarat C Panigrahi, Bhubaneswar
Dr Devanand Mohapatra, Bhubaneswar
Dr Asutosh Mohapatra, Bhubaneswar
Dr Susant Sethi, Bhubaneswar
Dr S Shanmughanathan, Chennai
Gopala Bisoi, Bhubaneswar
Malaya Mukhi, Bhubaneswar

Author

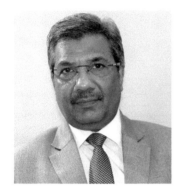

Dr Mohammad Ibrarullah is Senior Consultant in the Department of Surgical Gastroenterology, Apollo Hospitals, Bhubaneswar. Born in the state of Odisha, he obtained his graduate degree from SCB Medical College, Cuttack, Odisha, in 1985 and postgraduate degree in general surgery from JN Medical College, Aligarh, in 1988. He was associated with the Department of Surgical Gastroenterology, Sanjay Gandhi Postgraduate Institute of Medical Sciences, Lucknow, since its inception, and awarded a postdoctoral (MCh) degree in the super-specialty in 1995. The same year, he was selected as the "Travel Scholar of the International Society of Surgery Foundation" by the International Society of Surgery, USA. He has been a national faculty member in various academic forums and has contributed articles and research papers in several national and international journals and books.

Techniques of UGI endoscopy and normal anatomy

Preparation for endoscopy

Informed consent and counseling: The patient should be clearly informed about the procedure and the likely discomfort he may experience. It should be explained that his cooperation will make the procedure easier and quicker.

Overnight fasting: Routine endoscopy is usually performed in the morning hours after overnight fasting. Coating agents like antacids or colored medications should be clearly withheld. In case of obstructed stomach, prior nasogastric intubation and lavage should be performed to clear the gastric residue.

Sedation and anesthesia: For routine UGI endoscopy, we use only topical pharyngeal anesthetics such as lignocaine viscous or spray. Sedation, in the form of intravenous Midazolam, is occasionally used in children. For therapeutic endoscopy, such as foreign body removal, stent placement etc., it is our practice to use intravenous propofol anesthesia with or without endotracheal intubation.

Endotracheal intubation and monitoring: Endoscopy in a comatose or irritable patient is fraught with the risk of aspiration, hypoxia and "bite" damage to the endoscope. It is our practice to use prior endotracheal intubation and also monitor the vital parameters during the procedure.

Instrument check: Prior to endoscopy, it is good practice to check the instrument, including the light source, suction channel, airflow and display panel for any malfunction.

Position of the patient: Diagnostic endoscopy is always performed in the left lateral position. Occasionally, in a patient with upper GI bleeding, it may be necessary to examine the patient in the right lateral position. This is to displace the fundal blood pool that may obscure the bleeding lesion.

Antibiotic prophylaxis: Antibiotic prophylaxis is not indicated for diagnostic endoscopy. Current recommendations by the American Society for Gastrointestinal Endoscopy (ASGE) exclude even conditions such as valvular heart disease, prosthetic valves, synthetic vascular graft and prosthetic joints from the ambit of antibiotic prophylaxis. The few indications for antibiotic prophylaxis are therapeutic endoscopy for cirrhosis with acute variceal bleeding, cyst drainage and in patients with established GI tract infection who have the above listed cardiovascular status.

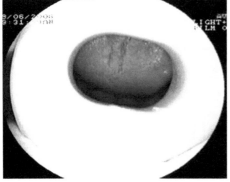

The mouth guard is held between the teeth. It is further supported by the index and middle finger of the endoscopy assistant. Alternatively, an elastic band attached to the mouth guard can be used to keep it steady.

Figure 1.1 The mouth guard.

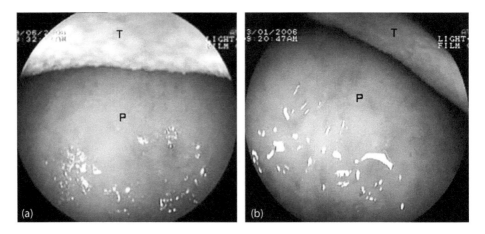

Figure 1.2 View as the endoscope enters the oral cavity. (a, b) Dorsum of the tongue (T) and hard palate (P).

The tip of the endoscope is slightly bent to fit the contour of the tongue. It is gently advanced over the base of the tongue towards the pharynx.

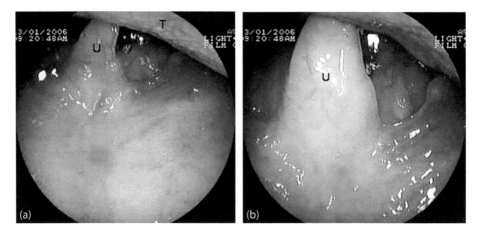

Figure 1.3 (a, b) Uvula (U) and the base of the tongue (T).

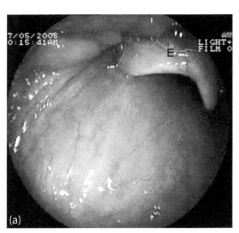
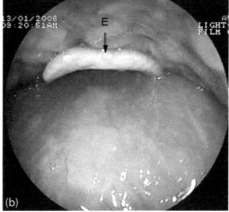

Figure 1.4 **(a, b)** Epiglottis (E).

The epiglottis (E) is seen as the pharynx is entered.

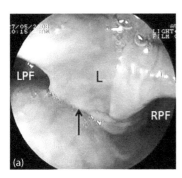
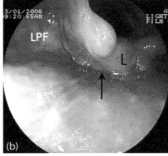
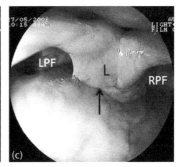

Figure 1.5 **(a–c)** The laryngo-pharynx. Larynx (L) and both pyriform fossae (RPF, LPF). The arrow points to the esophageal inlet.

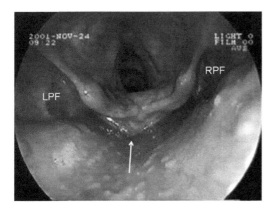

As the scope passes below the epiglottis, the larynx and both pyriform fossae come into view. The scope is kept in the midline at the esophageal inlet (arrow in Figures 1.5 & 1.6) and the patient is asked to take swallows. No undue force should be applied at this stage. Entry into the esophagus should be a voluntary effort supplemented by a gentle push by the endoscopist.

Figure 1.6 Larynx, right and left pyriform fossae (RPF & LPF, respectively) and the esophageal inlet (arrow).

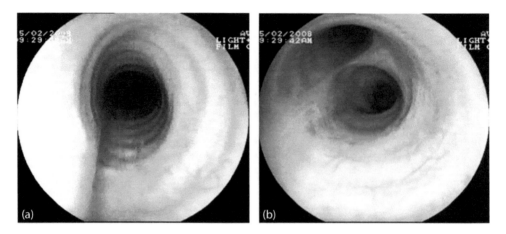

Figure 1.7 **(a)** Concentric rings of trachea. **(b)** Tracheal bifurcation.

While negotiating the esophageal inlet, such an appearance indicates passage of the endoscope into the trachea. The patient becomes restless and starts coughing violently. Withdraw the endoscope at once. Reassure the patient and retry entering the esophagus after a while.

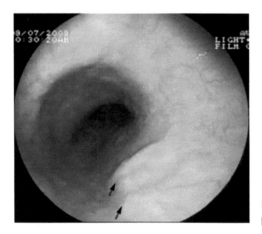

Figure 1.8 Tracheal impression (arrows) in the proximal esophagus.

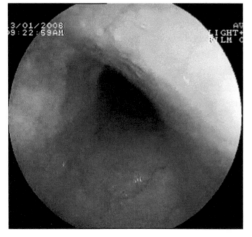

Esophageal mucosa is essentially featureless. The tracheal impression can be seen in the proximal esophagus. Aortic impression and pulsation can be observed in the mid-esophagus.

Figure 1.9 Mid-esophagus.

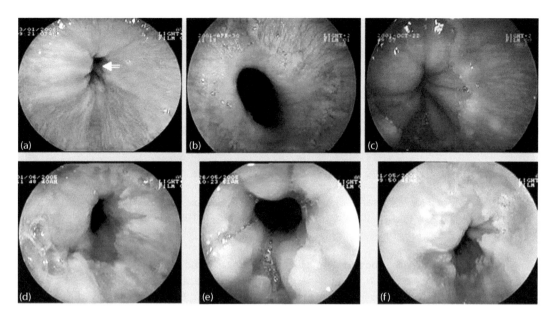

Figure 1.10 (a–f) Z line: The squamocolumnar (gastroesophageal) junction.

Z line represents the junction of pale squamous epithelium of the esophagus with the pink columnar epithelium of the stomach. This also marks the most proximal extent of the gastric folds. The junction may not be quite apparent when it lies at the level of diaphragmatic indentation (arrow in Figure 1.10a). In most cases, however, the junction can be made out clearly.

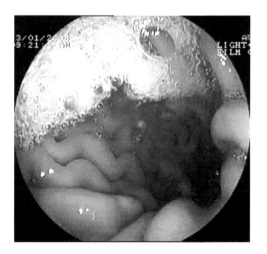

Figure 1.11 Gastric body.

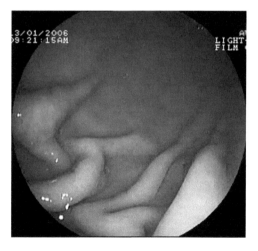

Figure 1.12 Junction of gastric body and antrum.

After crossing the GE junction, the tip of the endoscope is slightly angled up and to the right. As the stomach is inflated, a tunnel (Figure 1.11) becomes apparent. The roof and the base of the tunnel represent the lesser and greater curvatures, respectively. The endoscope is maintained close to the lesser curvature and gradually pushed forward. The mucosal rugosity in the gastric body turns flat marking the beginning of the antrum.

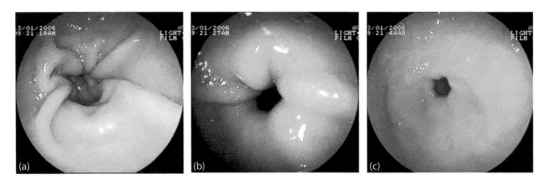

Figure 1.13 Pylorus. (a) Mucosal folds converging on the pylorus. (b) Mucosal folds around the pylorus partially flattened out. (c) Antral mucosa completely flattened out revealing the circular pylorus.

After inspecting the antrum, the endoscope is directed towards the pylorus. It is a common practice to cross the pylorus, examine D1, D2 and then come back to the antrum and complete examination of the remaining stomach. Crossing the pylorus is usually a frustrating experience for the beginner. In our practice, we advise the trainee endoscopist to use intravenous hyoscine bromide (Buscopan) to knock down gastric peristalsis, keep the pylorus in the center of vision, wait for the ring to open and then attempt to negotiate it. However, after a few endoscopies (usually 8–10), it ceases to be an issue and the endoscopist can cross the pylorus without much difficulty.

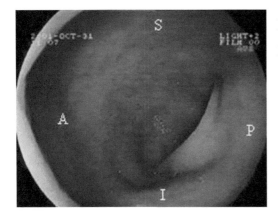

All the four walls of D1 are better visualized when the tip of the endoscope is placed at the pyloric ring (transpyloric view). Normally, the D1 mucosa is featureless.

Figure 1.14 Transpyloric view of the duodenal bulb (D1). The anterior wall (A), posterior wall (P), superior wall (S) and inferior wall (I).

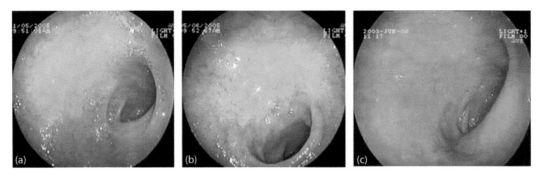

Figure 1.15 (a–c) Duodenal bulb.

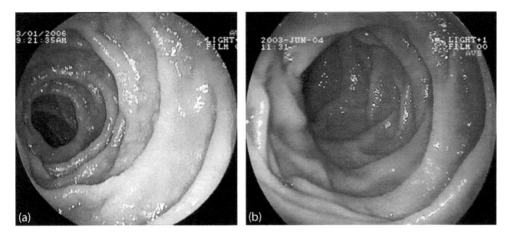

Figure 1.16 **(a, b)** The second part of the duodenum (D2) is marked by the circular mucosal folds.

The tip of the endoscope is impacted at the apex of D1 and rotated up and right. This maneuver facilitates entry into D2. As the endoscope is withdrawn slightly, its tip slips further down into D3. The ampulla of Vater can be seen on the medial wall of D2. This is the distal extent of examination for routine UGI endoscopy.

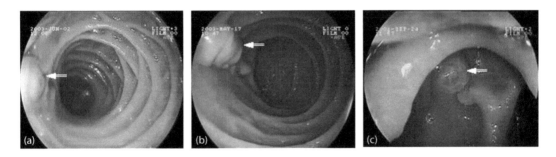

Figure 1.17 **(a–c)** Ampulla of Vater (arrow) seen on the medial wall of D2.

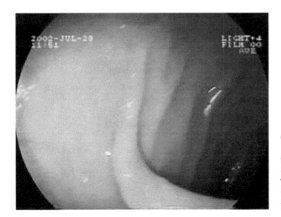

The endoscope is now gradually withdrawn, carefully examining all four walls of D2. The junction of D1-D2 is better inspected at this stage as the tip of the endoscope has a tendency to slip down during forward examination.

Figure 1.18 Junction of D1 and D2.

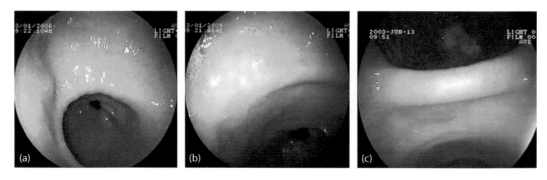

Figure 1.19 **(a, b)** Antrum and pylorus. **(c)** Incisura angularis.

The endoscope is withdrawn into the antrum for examination of the remaining part of stomach. The tip of the endoscope is flexed up, bringing into view the incisura angularis. In this position, the endoscope is gradually withdrawn maintaining constant insufflation and slight rotation to the left. By this retroflexion, or "J" maneuver, the entire lesser curvature can be inspected as the fundus is approached.

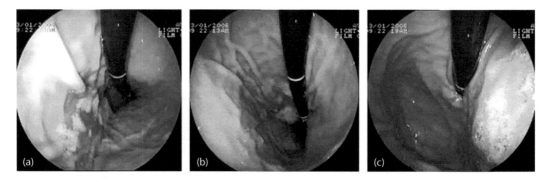

Figure 1.20 **(a–c)** The gastric fundus, as it appears during retroflexion ("J" maneuver).

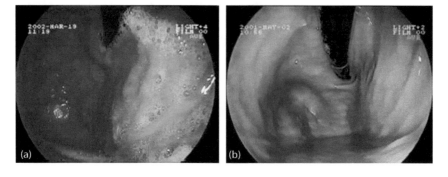

Figure 1.21 **(a, b)** The gastric fundus and the GE junction.

Fluid tends to accumulate in the fundus as this is the most dependent part of the stomach during endoscopy. This "fundic pool" needs to be sucked out to have a clear view of the mucosa. The GE junction can be inspected from a close proximity by withdrawing and rotating the endoscope further. Normally, the GE junction should appear snug around the shaft of the endoscope. This completes the examination of the upper GI tract. The tip of the endoscope is rotated to the normal position, air in the stomach is sucked out and the instrument is withdrawn.

2

Esophageal webs, rings and strictures

Webs and rings commonly present with dysphagia. Their appearance ranges from a thin, fibrous membrane partially occluding the lumen, to well-formed, concentric, fleshy rings having all three layers (i.e., mucosa, submucosa and muscles).

ETIOLOGY

- Congenital
- Iron-deficiency anemia (Plummer–Vinson syndrome, Paterson–Kelly syndrome)
- Eosinophilic gastroenteritis
- GERD
- Tropical sprue
- Autoimmune disorders
- Idiopathic

Diagnosis of postcricoid webs/strictures may be technically difficult as these are obscured by the cricopharyngeus. In such a situation, failure to intubate beyond the cricopharyngeus is often attributed by an inexperienced endoscopist to his own inefficiency or an uncooperative patient. When suspected, the tip of the endoscope should be placed at the esophageal inlet and the patient is asked to take swallows. The obstruction will be apparent when the cricopharyngeus opens transiently during deglutition.

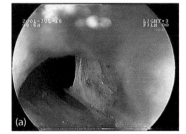
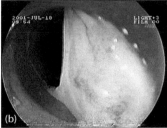
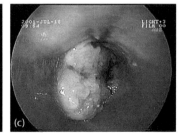

Figure 2.1 **(a, b)** Postcricoid web. The membrane occluding nearly two-thirds of the lumen was evident just below the cricopharyngeal sphincter. The patient presented with anemia and worsening of long-standing dysphagia. This could be explained as the endoscope was advanced further. **(c)** Squamous cell carcinoma in the distal esophagus in the same patient.

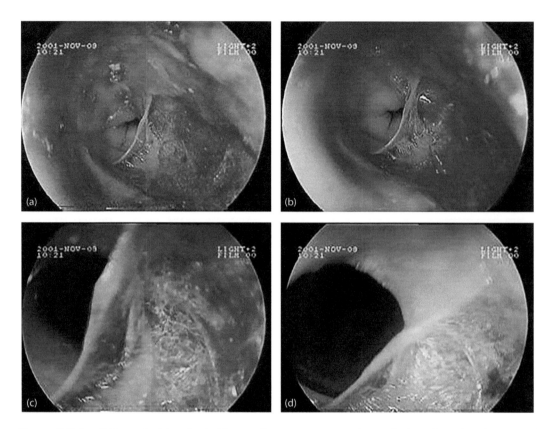

Figure 2.2 (a–d) Postcricoid web. A thin, semitransparent membrane below the cricopharyngeal sphincter. The membrane could be ruptured by gentle pushing with the tip of the endoscope.

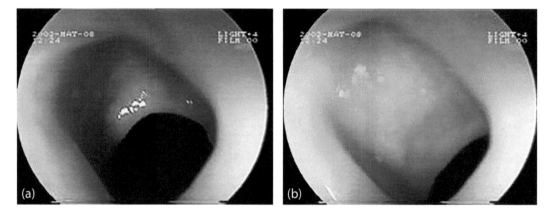

Figure 2.3 (a, b) Postcricoid web. A fleshy, concentric ring just below the cricopharyngeal sphincter in an elderly woman who presented with anemia and mild dysphagia.

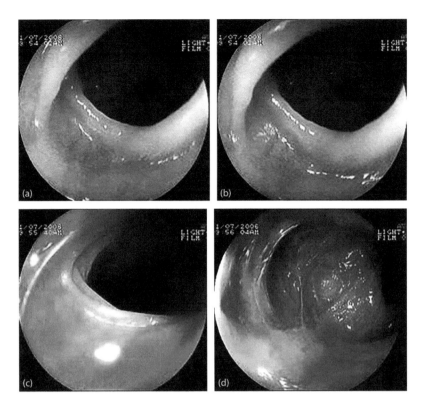

Figure 2.4 **(a–c)** Postcricoid rings. Multiple semicircular rings just below the cricopharyngeal sphincter in a middle-aged man who presented with dysphagia. **(d)** Mucosal tear following dilatation of the segment.

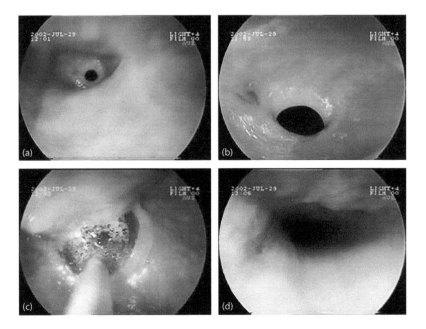

Figure 2.5 **(a, b)** Postcricoid ring. A fleshy, concentric ring just below the cricopharyngeal sphincter in a middle-aged woman who presented with mild dysphagia. **(c, d)** The ring was dilated with an endoscopic balloon.

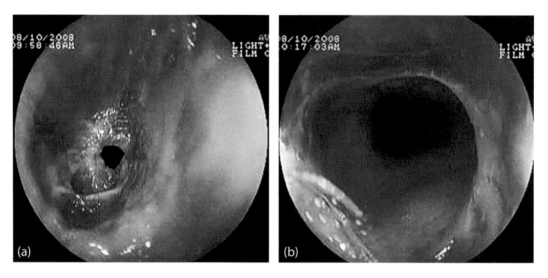

Figure 2.6 **(a)** Postcricoid membranous stricture in a middle-aged woman who presented with long-standing dysphagia. **(b)** The affected segment after dilatation.

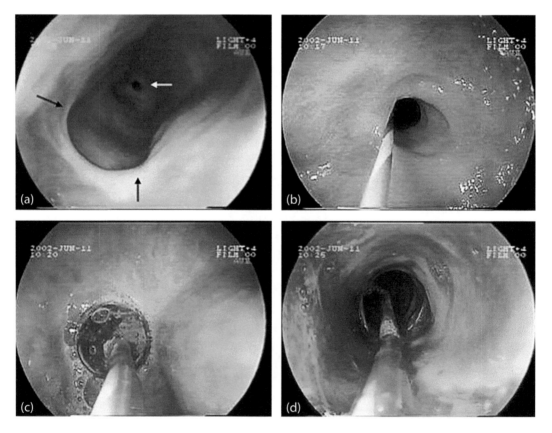

Figure 2.7 **(a)** Benign stricture in a young woman. Note the proximal one (black arrows) in the mid-esophagus is wider and passable; the distal one (white arrow) is tighter. **(b)** A guidewire across the distal stricture. **(c)** The distal stricture is being dilated with a balloon. **(d)** The same after dilatation.

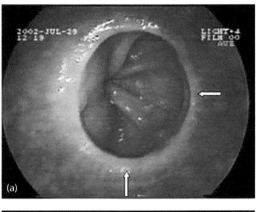

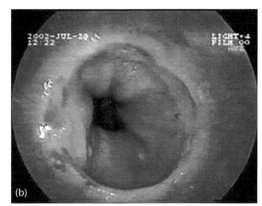

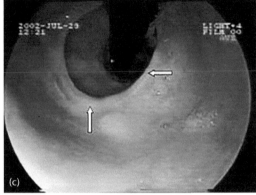

Figure 2.8 (a, b) Schatzki's ring. (c) Same as seen on retroflexion of endoscope. Note the associated hiatal hernia.

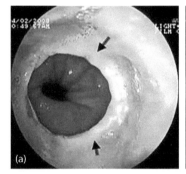

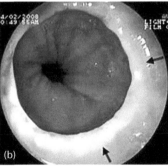

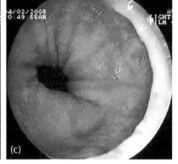

Figure 2.9 (a–c) Schatzki's ring (arrows) with sliding hiatal hernia.

Schatzki's ring is a well-demarcated circumferential stricture located at the squamocolumnar junction comprising mucosa and submucosa. This ring is more often an incidental finding, and hiatal hernia is a universal accompaniment. Dysphagia, if present (when the ring is critically narrowed), responds well to dilatation.

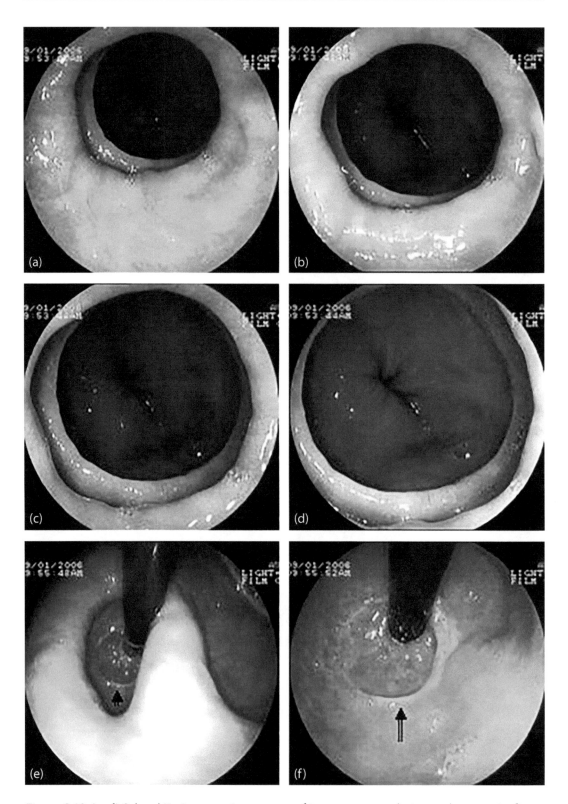

Figure 2.10 (a–d) Schatzki's ring at various stages of its appearance during endoscopy. (e, f) The ring (arrow) inside the hiatal sac as seen on retroflexion.

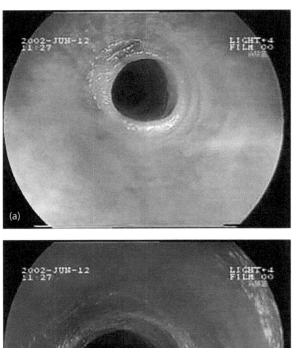

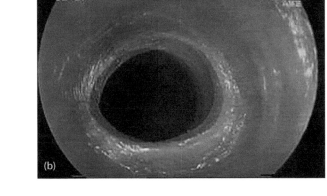

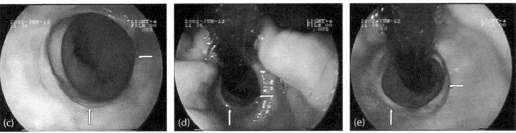

Figure 2.11 Postcricoid ring and Schatzki's ring. (a) Postcricoid ring in an elderly woman presenting with mild dysphagia. (b) Close-up view of the same. (c) Schatzki's ring (arrow) with hiatal hernia in the same patient. (d) The ring (arrow) as seen through the hiatal sac on retroflexion of the endoscope. (e) Close-up view of the same.

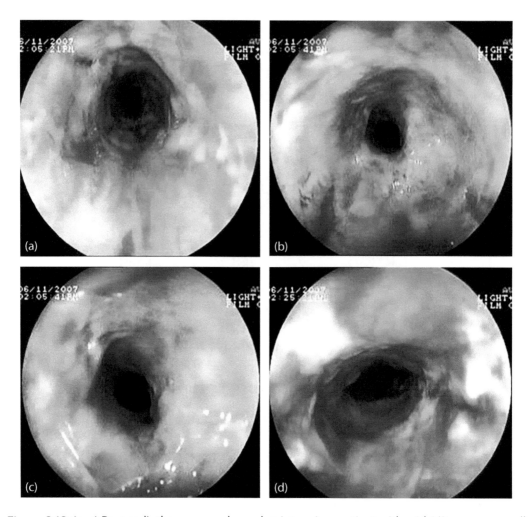

Figure 2.12 **(a–c)** Post-radiotherapy esophageal stricture in a patient with mid 1/3 squamous cell carcinoma. **(d)** Same after dilatation.

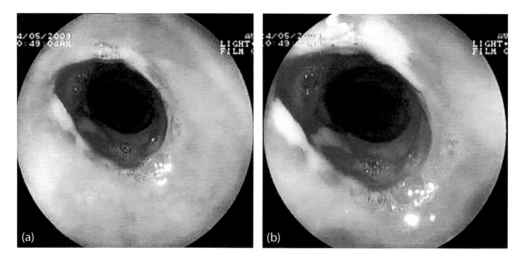

Figure 2.13 **(a, b)** Post-radiotherapy stricture in the mid-esophagus.

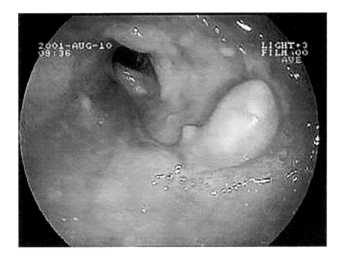

Figure 2.14 Post-sclerotherapy stricture at the lower end of esophagus. Esophageal varices were treated with intra- and paravariceal alcohol injection. Obliterated varix appear as mucosal tag.

Alcohol, in comparison with other sclerosants, has been associated with a higher incidence of stricture formation.

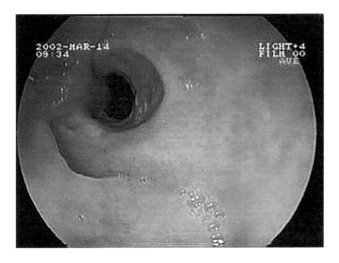

Figure 2.15 Post-sclerotherapy stricture at the lower end of esophagus.

Esophageal strictures following corrosive injury and peptic esophagitis have been presented elsewhere.

3

Hiatal hernia and gastroesophageal reflux disease (GERD)

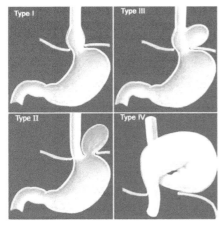

Figure 3.1 Classification of hiatal hernia.

CLASSIFICATION OF HIATAL HERNIA

Type I: Sliding hiatal hernia – cardia in chest
Type II: Paraesophageal hernia – GE junction in normal position, fundus in chest
Type III: Paraesophageal hernia – GE junction and fundus of stomach in chest
Type IV: Intrathoracic stomach ± volvulus

Type I and type III are the commonest and second commonest variants, respectively.

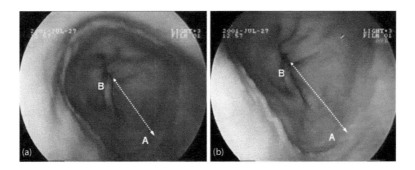

Figure 3.2 Sliding hiatal hernia.

SLIDING HIATAL HERNIA – ENDOSCOPIC DIAGNOSIS

- Distance between the squamocolumnar junction and the diaphragmatic indentation (A & B respectively in Figure 3.2) is >2 cm. Normally, it is <0.5 cm.
- On retroflexion, the diaphragmatic indentation (black arrows in Figure 3.3) is not snug around the endoscope. The "bell"-like appearance represents the hiatal sac. Gastric mucosa appears drawn into the hiatal sac.

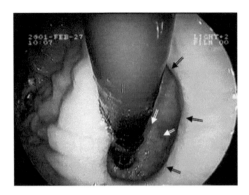

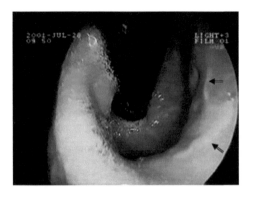

Figure 3.3 Sliding hiatal hernia; view on retroflexion. Note the diaphragmatic indentation (black arrows) and the squamocolumnar junction (white arrows).

Figure 3.4 Lax lower esophageal sphincter (LES); view on retroflexion. Note the squamocolumnar junction (arrows) is at the level of diaphragmatic indentation. This feature differentiates it from sliding hiatal hernia despite the similarity in appearance between the two.

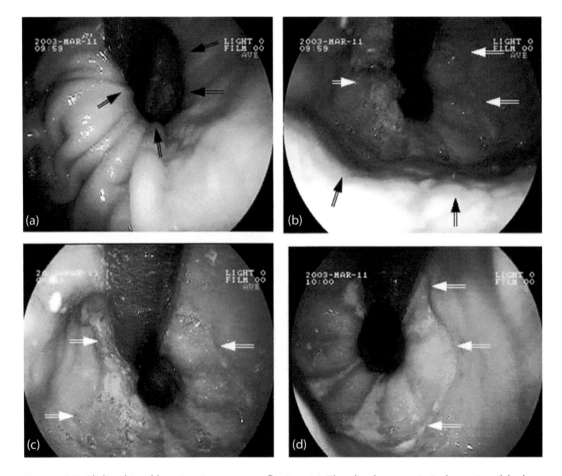

Figure 3.5 Sliding hiatal hernia; view on retroflexion. (a) The diaphragmatic indentation (black arrows) is not snug around the endoscope. The gastric mucosa has been pulled into the hiatal sac. (b, c) The squamocolumnar junction (white arrows) is above the diaphragmatic indentation. (d) Linear erosions in the esophageal mucosa stopping at the squamocolumnar junction.

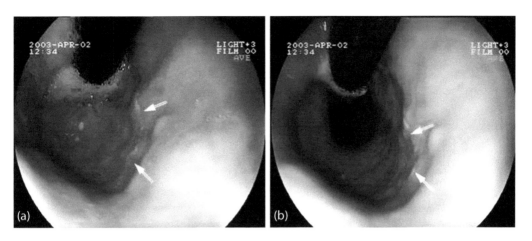

Figure 3.6 **(a, b)** Lax LES; View on retroflexion. Note the squamocolumnar junction (arrows) is almost coinciding with diaphragmatic indentation.

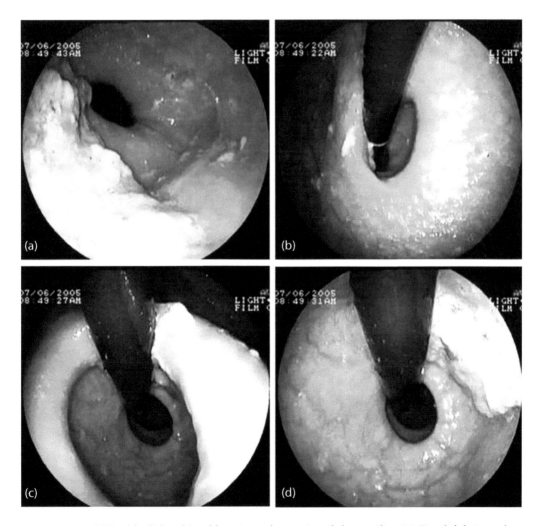

Figure 3.7 Lax LES with sliding hiatal hernia and associated dysmotility. **(a)** Food debris at the distal esophagus. The LES is open. **(b–d)** View on retroflexion.

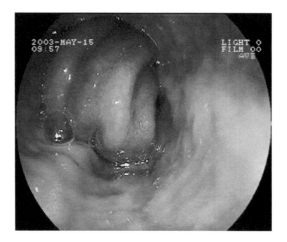

Figure 3.8 Gastric mucosal prolapse through lax LES.

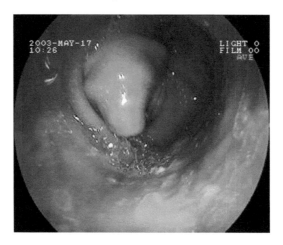

Figure 3.9 Sliding hiatal hernia and gastric mucosal prolapse.

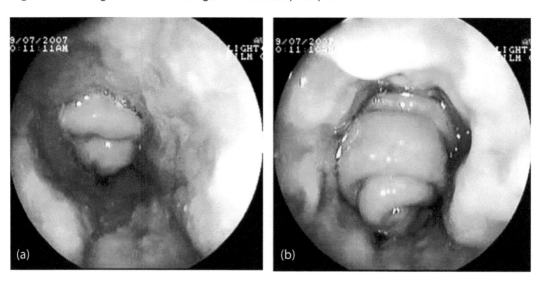

Figure 3.10 (a, b) Sliding hiatal hernia and gastric mucosal prolapse.

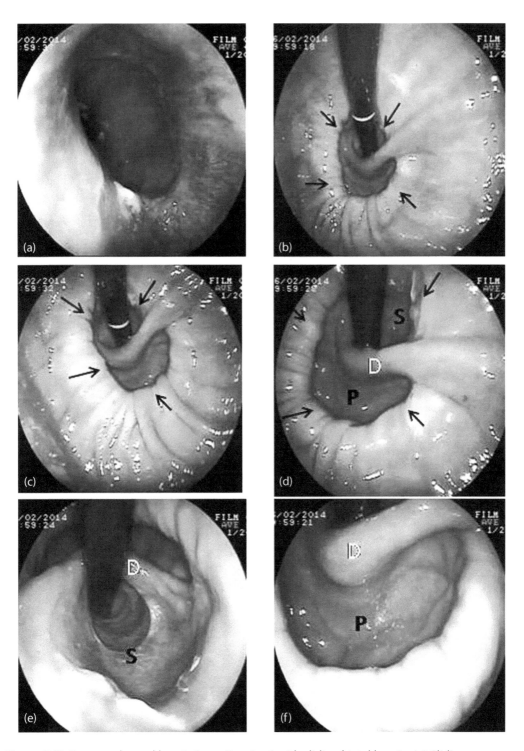

Figure 3.11 Paraesophageal hernia (type II variant) with sliding hiatal hernia. **(a)** Sliding component of hiatal hernia seen on forward view. **(b–d)** View on retroflexion. Note the diaphragmatic margin (arrows). Note the diaphragmatic bridge (D) between two hiatal sacs. **(e)** Close-up view of the sliding hernia sac (S) on retroflexion. Note the visible Z line and the lax LES through which the esophageal body could be seen. **(f)** Close-up view of the paraesophageal herniated fundus (P) on retroflexion.

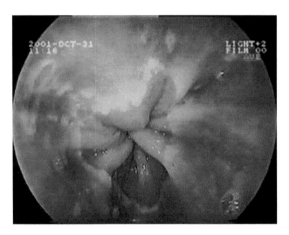

Figure 3.12 Oval erosions just above the Z line.

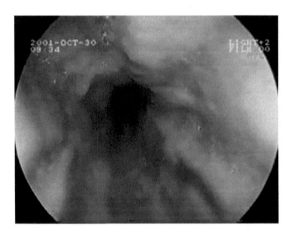

Figure 3.13 Reflux induced linear erosion.

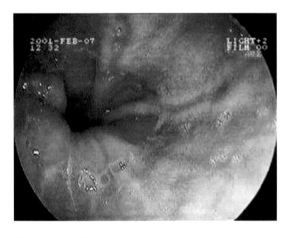

Figure 3.14 Linear erosion.

ENDOSCOPIC GRADING OF GERD

Savary Miller grading

Grade I

Oval or linear red patch situated above "Z" line, often along a dorsal fold, may be covered with whitish exudate. Occasionally many such lesions are present, but they are not confluent.

Grade II

The erosive and exudative mucosal lesions are confluent but not involving the entire circumference.

Grade III

Involvement of entire circumference but stricturing is absent.

Grade IV

Presence of stricture or longitudinal shortening and/or the development of columnar metaplasia.

Handbook & Atlas of Endoscopy, Solothurn, Schweiz: Gasman 1978

Los Angeles grading

Grade A

One or more mucosal break(s) no longer than 5 mm, that does not extend between the top of two mucosal folds.

Grade B

One or more mucosal break(s) >5 mm long, not extending between the tops of two mucosal folds.

Grade C

One or more mucosal breaks between the top of two or more mucosal folds involving <75% of the circumference.

Grade D

One or more mucosal break(s) involving at least 75% of the esophageal circumference.

Gut 1999; 45:172

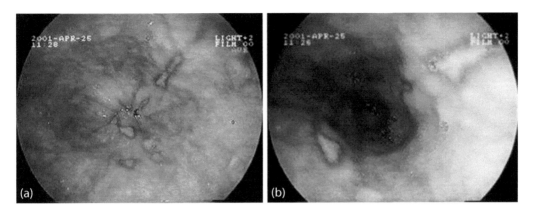

Figure 3.15 **(a, b)** Erosions in the distal esophagus.

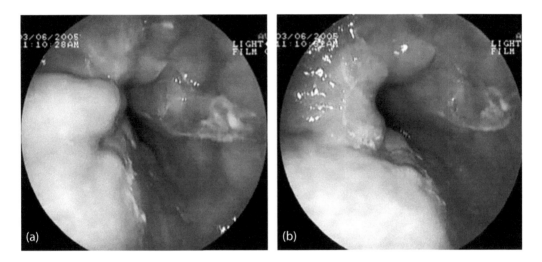

Figure 3.16 **(a, b)** Erosions and exudates at the GE junction.

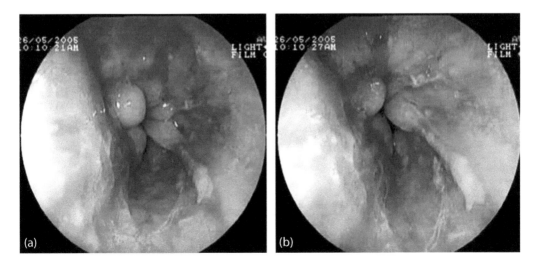

Figure 3.17 **(a, b)** Linear erosions at the GE junction.

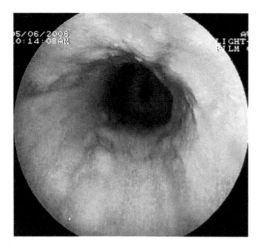

Figure 3.18 Erosions extending up to the mid-esophagus.

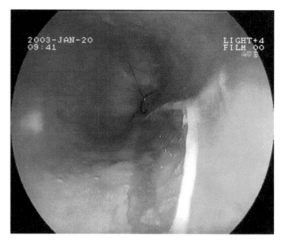

Figure 3.19 Erosion extending proximally.

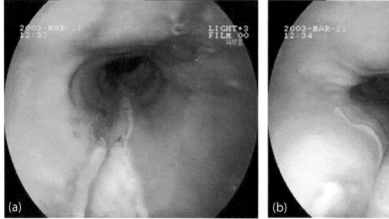
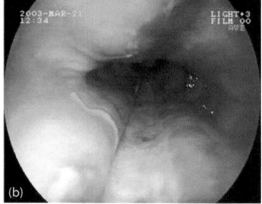

Figure 3.20 (a, b) Linear ulcer extending from the GE junction to the proximal esophagus.

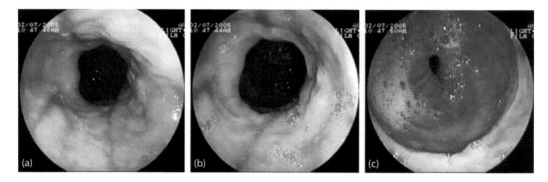

Figure 3.21 (a, b) Linear erosions. (c) Sliding hiatal hernia in the same patient.

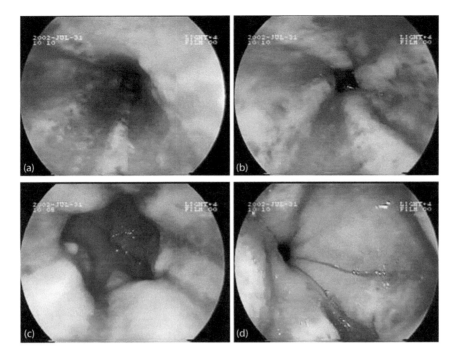

Figure 3.22 (a–d) Erosions extending up to the squamocolumnar junction.

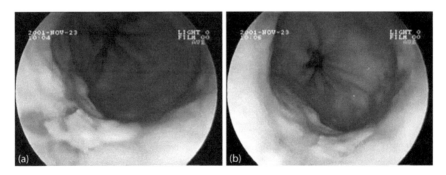

Figure 3.23 (a, b) Sliding hiatal hernia. An ulcer at the six-o'clock position proximal to the squamocolumnar junction.

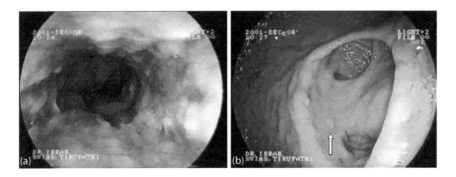

Figure 3.24 (a) Extensive ulceration involving the distal esophageal mucosa.
(b) Gastrojejunostomy stoma in the same patient showing small erosion (arrow).

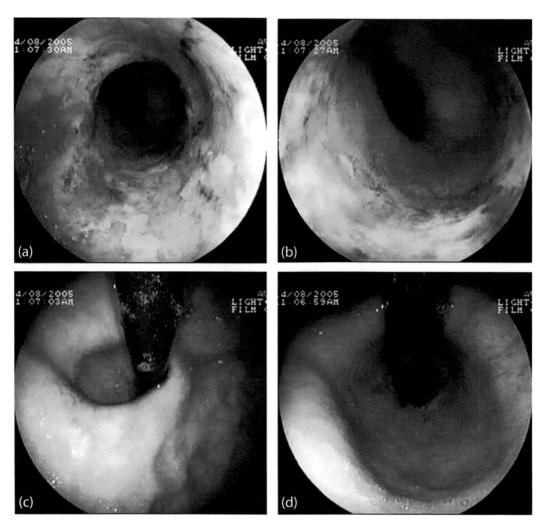

Figure 3.25 (a, b) Esophagitis with sliding hiatal hernia. (c, d) View of the hernial sac on retroflexion.

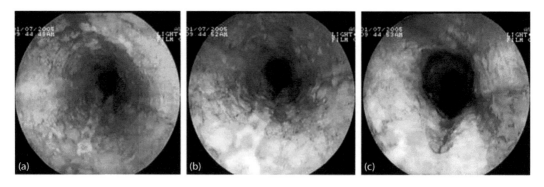

Figure 3.26 (a–c) Extensive esophageal involvement in GERD.

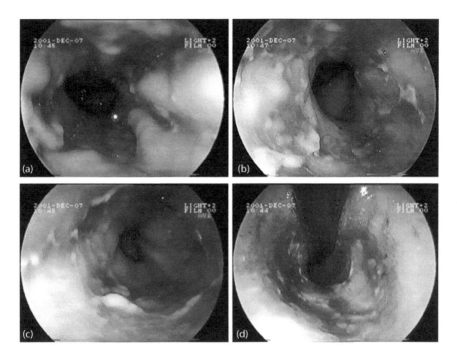

Figure 3.27 (a–c) Erosive esophagitis with sliding hiatal hernia. (d) View on retroflexion.

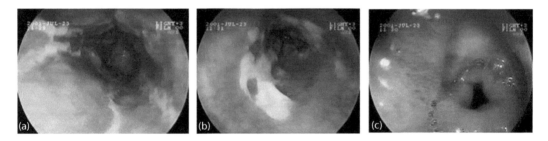

Figure 3.28 (a, b) Esophagitis with overlying exudates extending up to the mid-esophagus. (c) A giant duodenal ulcer in the same patient.

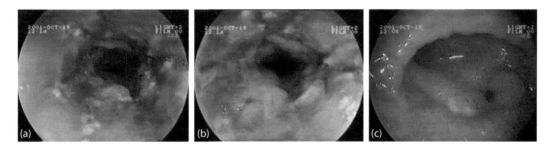

Figure 3.29 (a, b) Erosive esophagitis. (c) Prepyloric ulcer with pseudo diverticulum in the same patient.

Concomitant peptic ulcer is not unusual in patients suffering from severe esophagitis. Hyperacidity is found in 28% of patients suffering from GERD.

Archives of Surgery 1989:124; 937.

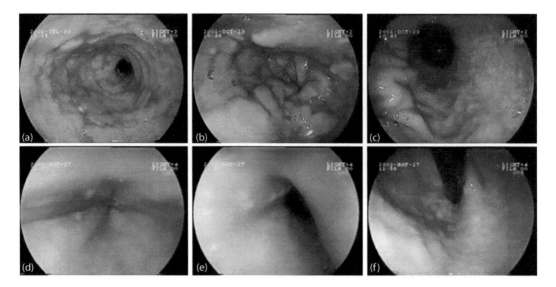

Figure 3.30 (a, b) Bile reflux esophagitis. Mucosal changes at the lower end of esophagus in a patient who had undergone gastrojejunostomy about 10 years back. (c) Hiatal hernia in the same patient. He was treated with Roux-en-Y conversion and partial fundoplication. (d, e) Normal appearing esophageal mucosa, six months after the surgery. (f) Consequent upon fundoplication, on retroflexion the gastric mucosa is seen tightly gripping the endoscope at the cardia.

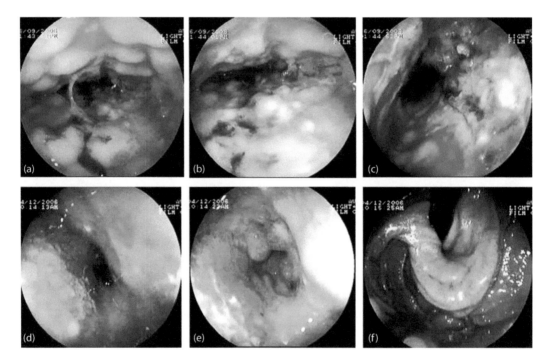

Figure 3.31 (a–c) Extensive ulceration involving distal esophagus. The patient underwent Nissen's fundoplication. (d, e) Endoscopy three months after surgery showing healed esophageal ulcers. (f) Retroflexed view of the cardia subsequent to fundoplication.

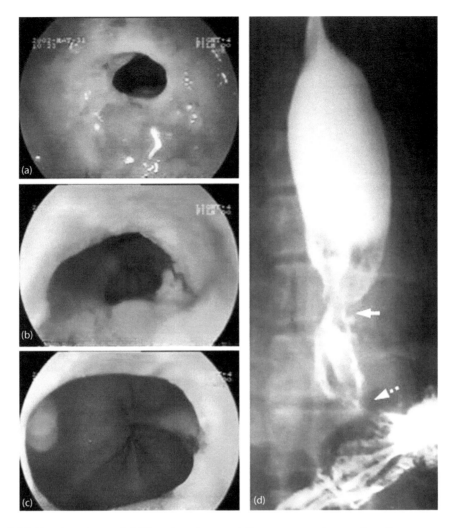

Figure 3.32 Peptic stricture (a) Fibrotic stricture at the squamocolumnar junction.
(b, c) Sliding hiatal hernia visible through the stricture. (d) Barium contrast study, in the same patient, showing stricture (arrow) at the distal esophagus and proximal dilatation. Note the diaphragmatic indentation (broken arrow) and the intervening hiatal sac.

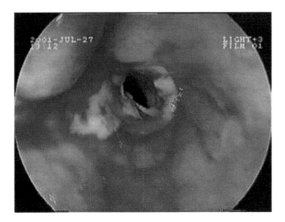

Figure 3.33 Peptic stricture in distal esophagus.

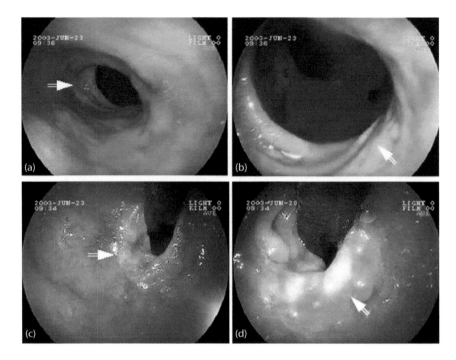

Figure 3.34 (a, b) Peptic stricture (arrow) and sliding hiatal hernia. (c, d) Close-up view of the stricture (arrow) on retroflexion showing fibrosis and nodularity.

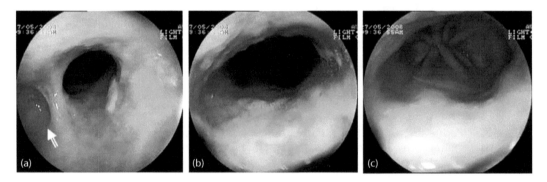

Figure 3.35 (a) Peptic stricture involving distal esophagus. Note the diverticulum (arrow) proximal to the stricture. (b, c) Sliding hiatal hernia in the same patient.

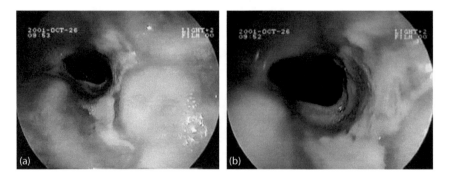

Figure 3.36 (a, b) Peptic stricture and esophageal ulcers.

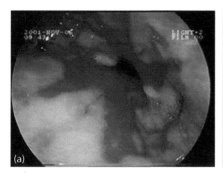
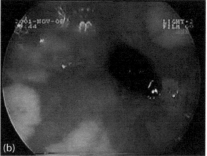

Figure 3.37 **(a, b)** Barrett's esophagus; flame-shaped extension of columnar epithelium into the esophagus.

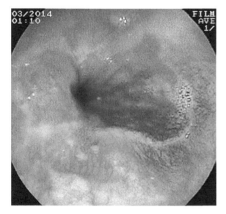

Figure 3.38 Short-segment Barrett's esophagus.

Barrett's esophagus is a known complication of GERD. It is characterized by a flame-shaped or finger-like extension of gastric columnar epithelium into the esophagus that typically displays intestinal metaplasia. Depending on the extent of involvement from the GE junction (defined as the upper limit of visible gastric fold), it is classified as short-segment (<3 cm) or long-segment (>3 cm) Barrett's. However, endoscopic maximal (M) and circumferential (C) extent of involvement in centimeters (Prague C & M criteria) is the current recommendation to document Barrett's esophagus. Because of its premalignant potential, four-quadrant biopsy, every 1–2 cm, and biopsy of any suspicious lesion have been recommended to detect dysplasia (Seattle protocol). Any visible lesion is characterized by the Paris classification. Mild and moderate dysplasia are treated with conventional anti-reflux treatment and kept under surveillance. High-grade dysplasia is treated by endoscopic ablation or surgical excision.

Gastroenterology 2011; 140 e 18
Gastrointest Endosc 2003; 58 (suppl): 3

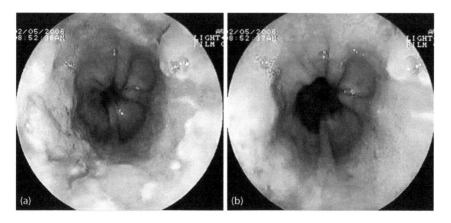

Figure 3.39 **(a, b)** Barrett's esophagus with sliding hiatal hernia.

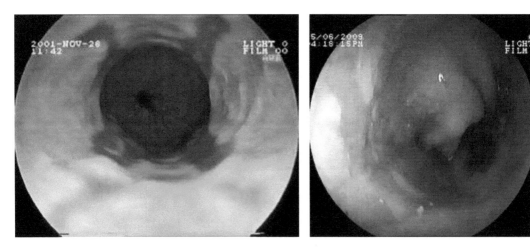

Figure 3.40 Barrett's esophagus.

Figure 3.41 Barrett's esophagus with sliding hiatal hernia.

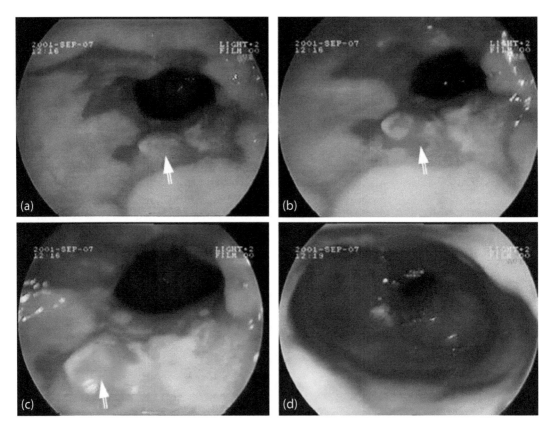

Figure 3.42 (a–c) Barrett's esophagus with dysplastic nodule (arrow). (d) Associated sliding hiatal hernia.

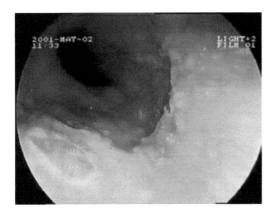

Figure 3.43 Barrett's mucosal island just above the Z line.

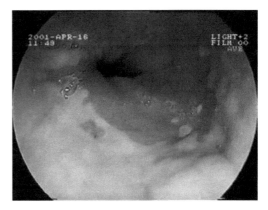

Figure 3.44 Barrett's esophagus. Note the finger-like projections as well as the island of columnar epithelium.

Table 3.1 Surveillance protocol for Barrett's esophagus

	ASGE	ACG	AGA
Screening	No Barrett's in suspected patients; no further screening required	Chronic GERD in age >50 y	White male >50 y with GERD
No dysplasia	Repeat endoscopy at 1 y and every 3rd year thereafter.	Repeat endoscopy and every 3rd year thereafter.	Repeat endoscopy and every 5 y thereafter
Low-grade dysplasia	Endoscopy every year	Endoscopy every year	Confirmed by two pathologists; endoscopy every year, otherwise every 2 y
High-grade dysplasia	Confirm biopsy; repeat endoscopy to exclude malignancy; endoscopic ablation/ surgical excision	Confirm biopsy; repeat endoscopy to exclude malignancy; endoscopic ablation/ surgical excision	Confirm biopsy; repeat endoscopy to exclude malignancy; intensive surveillance/ endoscopic ablation/ surgical excision

Abbreviations: ACG, American College of Gastroenterology; AGA, American Gastroenterological Association; ASGE, American Society for Gastrointestinal Endoscopy.

4

Motility disorders of the esophagus

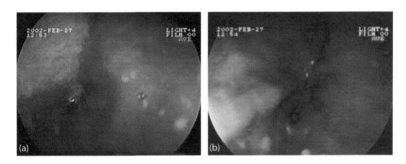

Figure 4.1 Achalasia cardia. **(a)** Dilated esophagus with food residue. **(b)** Non-relaxing lower esophageal sphincter (LES).

Endoscopic features of achalasia cardia include dilated and tortuous esophagus containing food residue. The LES initially offers resistance to the passage of the endoscope but "gives in" with mild force. The most important aspect of endoscopy, however, is detection of esophageal malignancy consequent upon long standing achalasia. It is also important to exclude secondary achalasia that arises from submucosal infiltration of the GE junction by adjacent malignancy. In the latter situation, considerable force is required to negotiate the endoscope across the LES. Once in the stomach, it is mandatory to retroflex and have an optimal view of the GE junction.

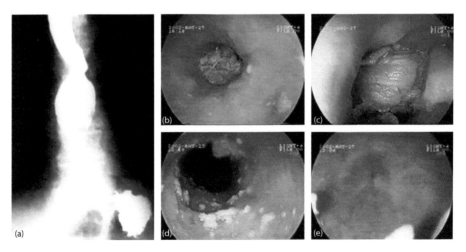

Figure 4.2 Achalasia cardia. **(a)** Barium-contrast study showing dilated and tortuous esophagus with "bird-beak" tapering. **(b, c)** Absent peristalsis resulting in food bolus impaction in the mid-esophagus. **(d)** Appearance of the distal esophagus after removal of the food bolus. **(e)** Non-relaxing LES.

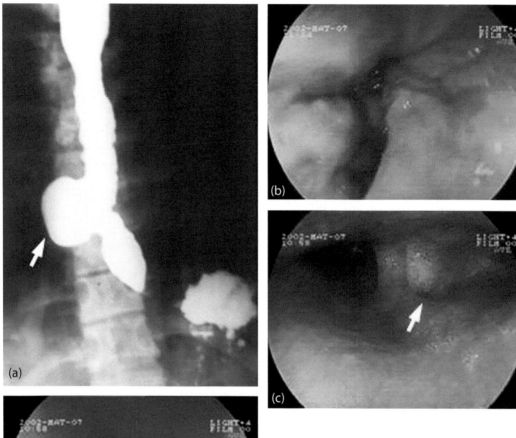

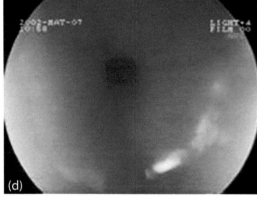

Figure 4.3 (a) Barium-contrast study showing dilated esophagus and epiphrenic diverticulum (arrow) in a young woman with achalasia cardia. (b) Dilated distal esophagus. (c) Diverticulum (arrow). (d) Non-relaxing LES.

5

Benign gastric ulcer

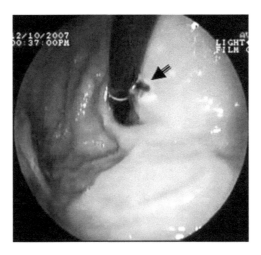

Figure 5.1 Ulcer just below the GE junction (arrow) seen on retroflexion.

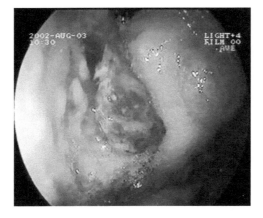

Figure 5.2 A giant ulcer below the GE junction seen on retroflexion.

Based on the location, gastric ulcers are categorized into four types. I: ulcer located on the lesser curve, II: associated with duodenal ulcer, III: prepyloric ulcer, IV: ulcer just below GE junction. Types II and III ulcers are associated with hyperacidity and behave as a duodenal ulcer with respect to symptomatology and treatment. Multiple ulcers are seen in association with NSAID use, chronic liver disease, heavy smokers or acute viral infection. Ulcers located high on lesser curvature are likely to be missed during forward passage of the endoscope and are best viewed on retroflexion.

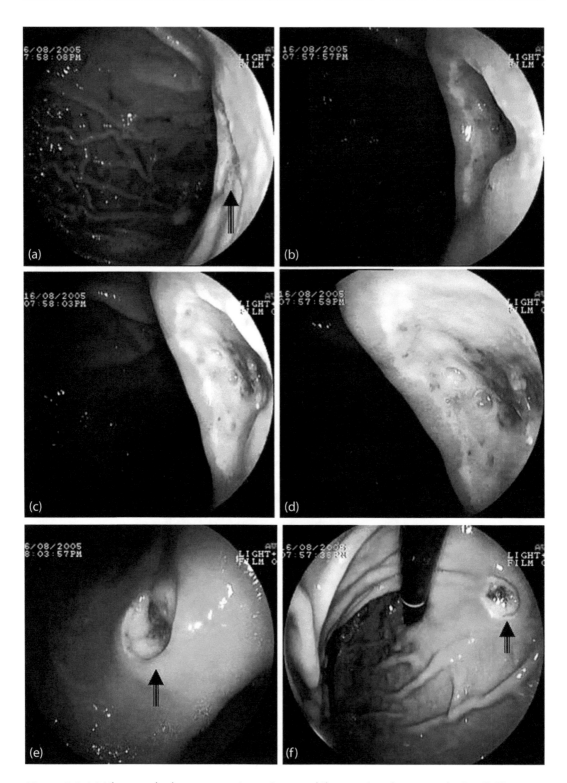

Figure 5.3 **(a)** Ulcer on the lesser curve (arrow) seen while entering the stomach. **(b–d)** Close-up view. **(e, f)** View on retroflexion. The patient presented with hematemesis and melena. Note the ulcer base showing stigmata of recent hemorrhage.

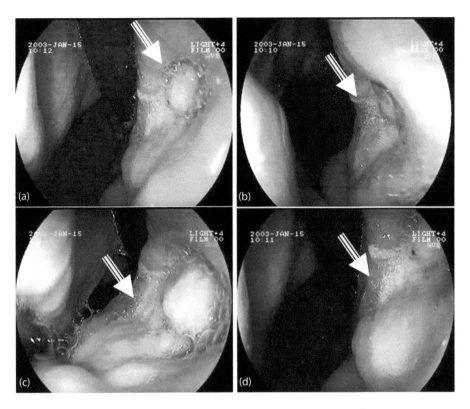

Figure 5.4 **(a–d)** Ulcer (arrow) high on the lesser curve as seen on retroflexion.

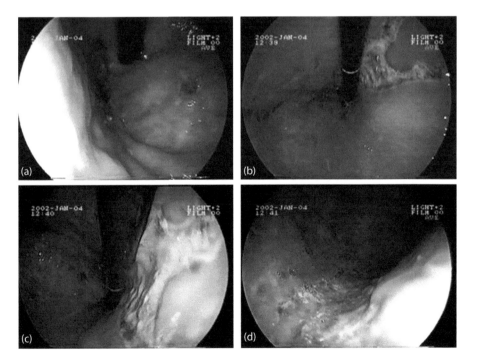

Figure 5.5 **(a–d)** Extensive ulceration involving proximal stomach. The patient, a known case of hepatitis, presented with hematemesis.

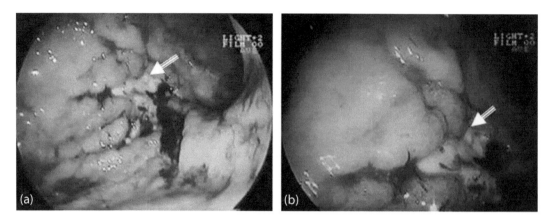

Figure 5.6 **(a, b)** Ulcer (arrow) in the body of the stomach. Such ulcer is likely to get hidden between the gastric folds. Adequate distention is required for its visualization.

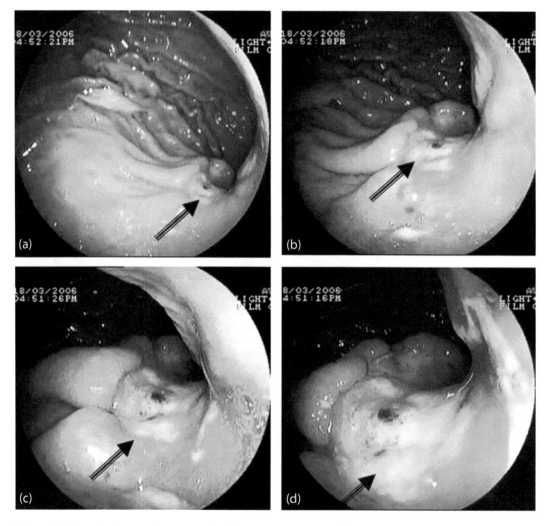

Figure 5.7 **(a–d)** Ulcer in the gastric body at various stages of its appearance during endoscopy. Note the flat red spot, suggesting a recent episode of bleeding.

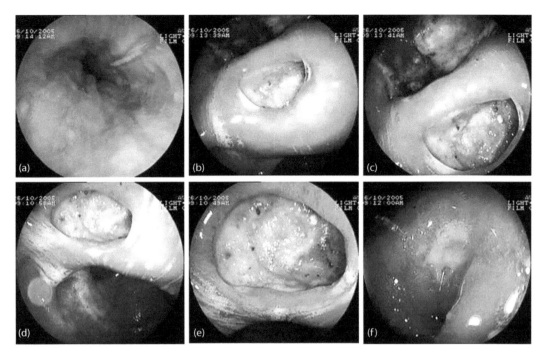

Figure 5.8 Endoscopy in an elderly man presenting with pain in the abdomen and retention vomiting. **(a)** Retention esophagitis. **(b–e)** A giant ulcer on the incisura. **(f)** Another superficial ulcer in the prepyloric region. The pylorus is deformed and narrowed. Note the gastric retention in (c).

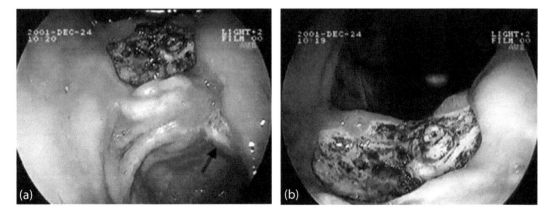

Figure 5.9 **(a, b)** Ulcer on the incisura. Note another small ulcer (arrow) below it.

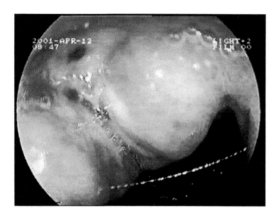

Figure 5.10 Ulcer on the incisura having flat red spots suggestive of recent hemorrhage.

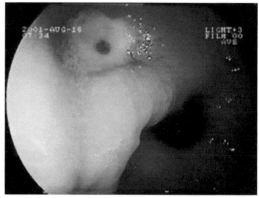

Figure 5.11 Ulcer on the incisura having flat red spot.

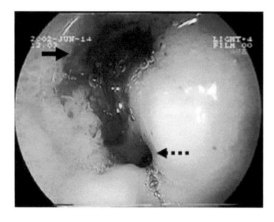

Figure 5.12 Ulcer (arrow) in the antrum hidden by the blood pool. Note the distorted pylorus (broken arrow).

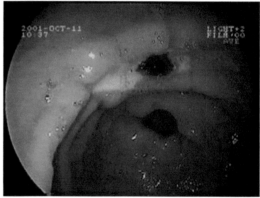

Figure 5.13 Ulcer on the incisura covered with acid hematin.

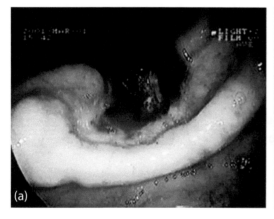

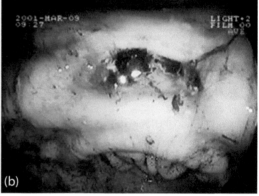

Figure 5.14 (a) Giant ulcer on the incisura with adherent clot. (b) Same ulcer one week later. Though partial healing was evident, the patient presented with bleeding recurrence.

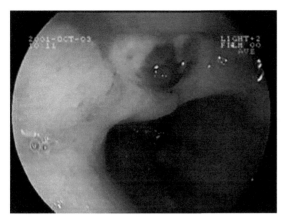

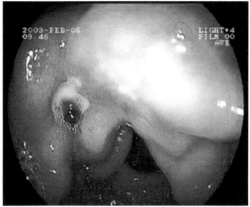

Figure 5.15 Oozing ulcer in the prepyloric antrum.

Figure 5.16 Ulcer in the prepyloric antrum having a visible vessel.

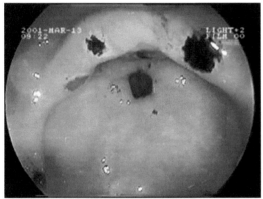

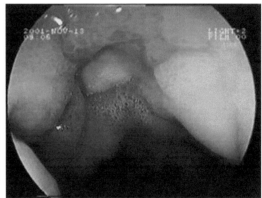

Figure 5.17 Multiple ulcers on the incisura covered with acid hematin.

Figure 5.18 Ulcer in the antrum with a clean base.

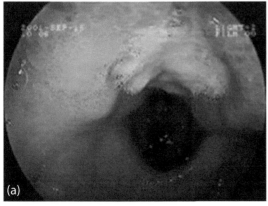

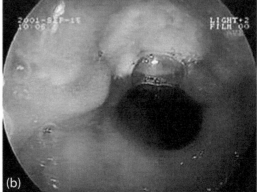

Figure 5.19 (a, b) Giant prepyloric ulcer.

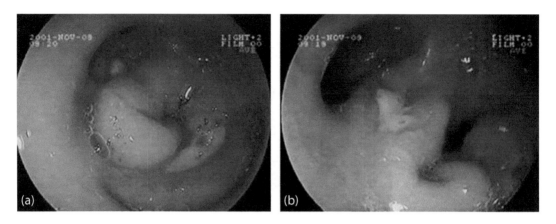

Figure 5.20 (a, b) Prepyloric ulcers, erosions and pseudodiverticulum.

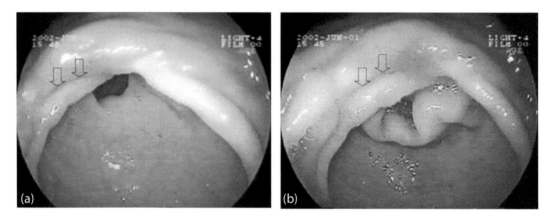

Figure 5.21 (a, b) Prepyloric ulcer (arrows) hidden in the mucosal folds. Unless the endoscopist is careful, such an ulcer may elude detection.

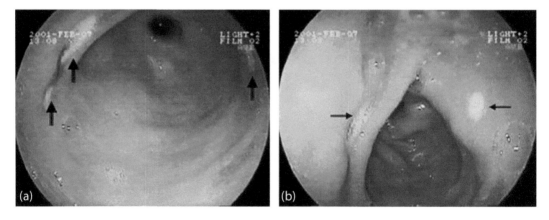

Figure 5.22 (a, b) Multiple prepyloric ulcers (arrows).

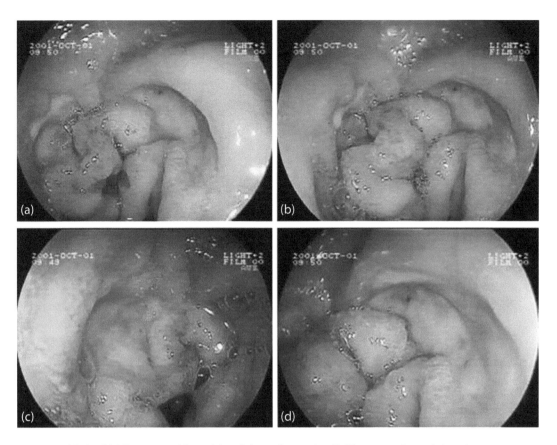

Figure 5.23 (a, b) Ulcers on either side of the pylorus. (c, d) Close-up view of the ulcers.

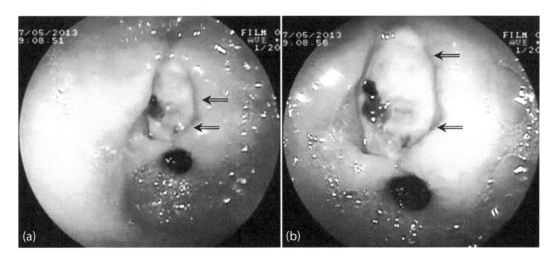

Figure 5.24 (a, b) Giant prepyloric ulcer showing recent evidence of bleeding.

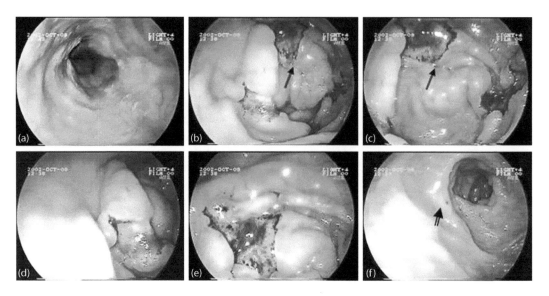

Figure 5.25 Multiple prepyloric ulcers in a patient with chronic liver disease. (a) Esophageal varices. (b, c) Giant ulcers around pylorus (arrow). (d) Close-up view of the ulcer at the nine-o'clock position. (e) Ulcer at the 12-o'clock position. (f) Superficial ulcer (arrow) in the duodenal bulb.

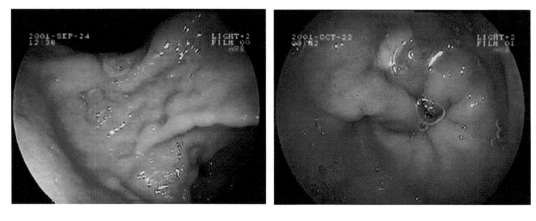

Figure 5.26 Multiple superficial ulcers in the antrum.

Figure 5.27 Prepyloric ulcer.

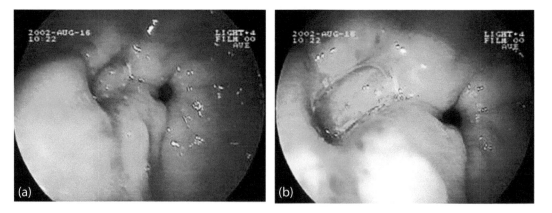

Figure 5.28 (a, b) Prepyloric ulcer.

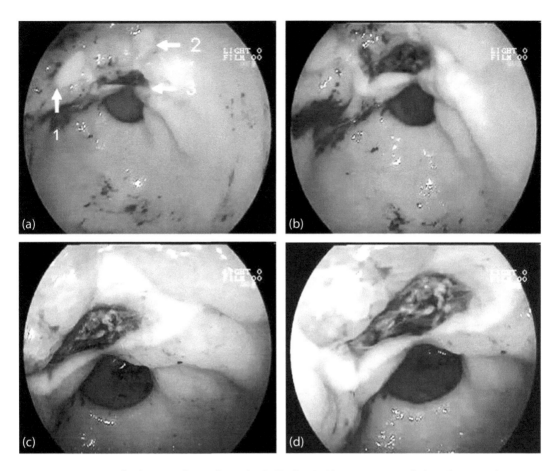

Figure 5.29 (a) Multiple prepyloric ulcers (1, 2, 3). (b–d) Close-up view of ulcer 3. Note the adherent clot suggestive of recent bleeding.

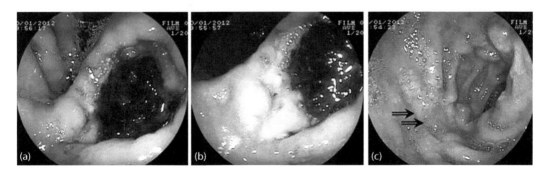

Figure 5.30 (a, b) Giant ulcer on incisura with adherent clot. (c) Concomitant duodenal ulcer (arrows).

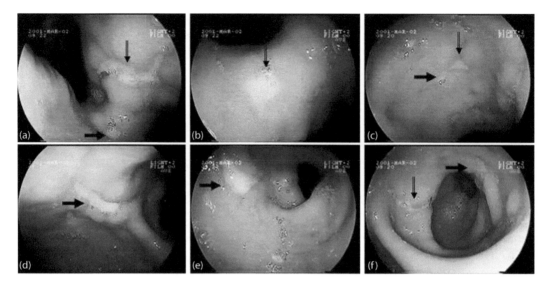

Figure 5.31 (a–f) Multiple ulcers (arrows) involving the antrum.

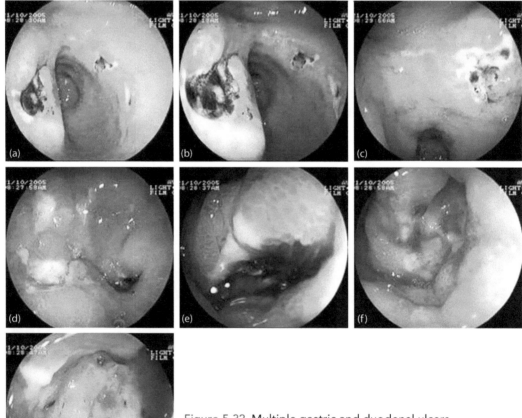

Figure 5.32 Multiple gastric and duodenal ulcers.
(a, b) Ulcers in the antrum. (c) Close-up view of the ulcer at the
two-o'clock position. (d) Ulcers in the prepyloric antrum. Note
the deformed pylorus and the duodenal ulcer seen through
it. (e) The duodenal ulcer appearing black due to presence of
acid hematin. (f, g) Close-up view of the duodenal ulcer.

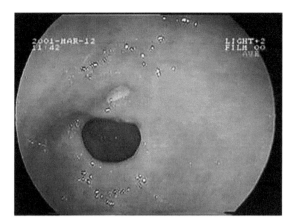

Figure 5.33 Prepyloric ulcer.

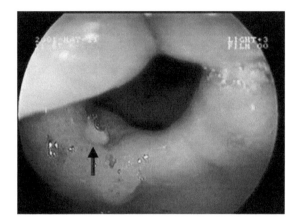

Figure 5.34 Pyloric channel ulcer (arrow).

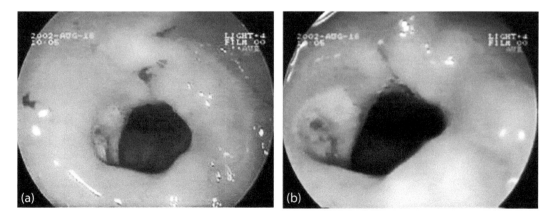

Figure 5.35 **(a, b)** Pyloric channel ulcer with evidence of recent bleeding.

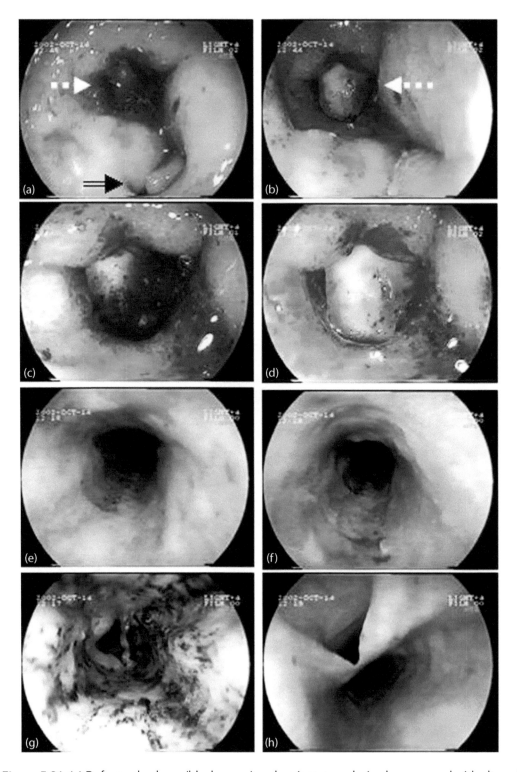

Figure 5.36 (a) Deformed pylorus (black arrow) and a giant prepyloric ulcer covered with altered blood (white arrow). (b–d) Close-up view of the same ulcer (white arrow) after the blood was cleaned. (e–g) Severe reflux esophagitis in the same patient. Entire esophagus covered with thick exudates. (h) The exudates forming a membrane in the upper esophagus.

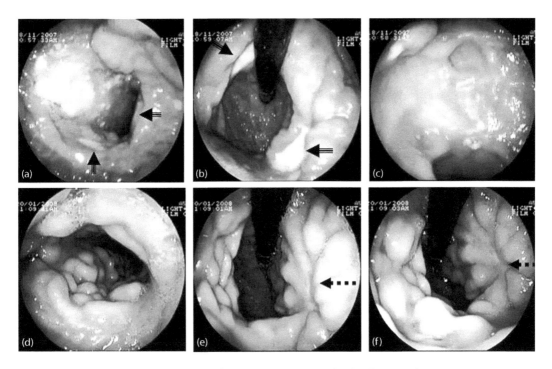

Figure 5.37 Hour-glass contracture of the stomach. **(a)** Multiple ulcers with cicatrization (arrows) causing circumferential narrowing in the gastric body. **(b)** Ulcers (arrows) are better seen on retroflexion. **(c)** Antrum, relatively healthy. **(d–f)** Ulcer healing and scarring (broken arrow) evident after treatment with proton pump inhibitors for eight weeks. Note the mucosal hypertrophy that could have resulted from obstruction as well as hyperacidity. The patient was a chronic smoker.

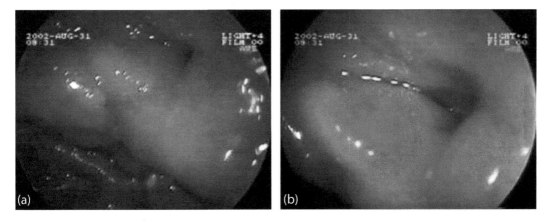

Figure 5.38 **(a, b)** Benign gastric outlet obstruction. Scarred and stenotic pylorus consequent upon ulcer healing.

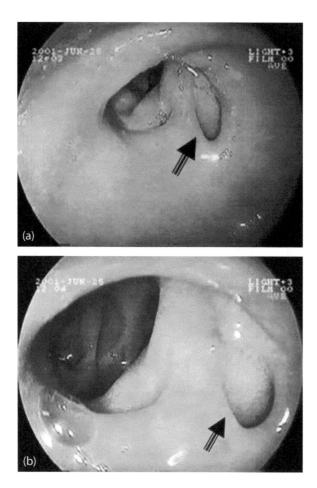

Figure 5.39 (a, b) Deformed pylorus with prepyloric pseudodiverticulum (arrow). Deformed duodenal bulb can be seen through the pyloric ring.

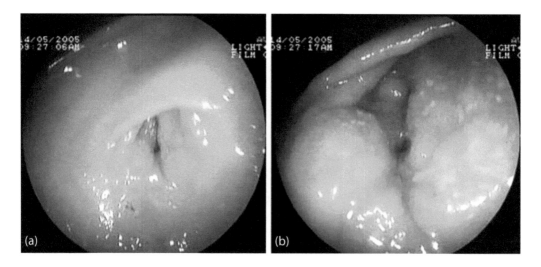

Figure 5.40 (a, b) Deformed and narrowed pylorus following ulcer healing.

6

Chronic duodenal ulcer

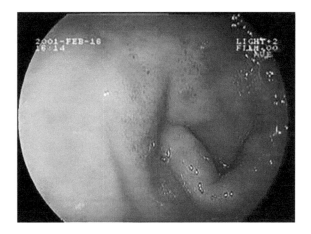

Figure 6.1 Duodenitis. Erythematous patches involving duodenal bulb (D1).

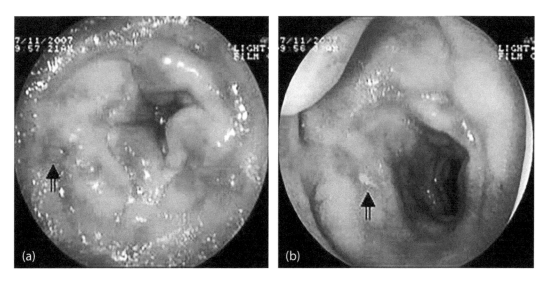

Figure 6.2 **(a, b)** Duodenitis with superficial ulcer (arrow) in D1.

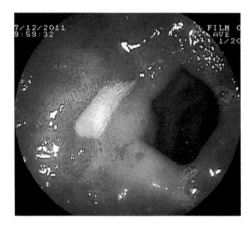

Figure 6.3 An active ulcer on the anterior wall of D1.

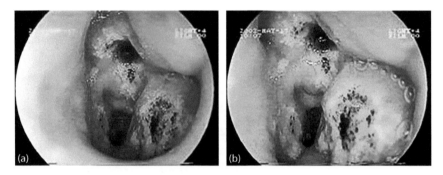

Figure 6.4 **(a, b)** Deformed duodenal bulb, multiple superficial ulcers and pseudodiverticula.

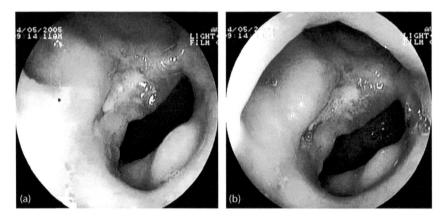

Figure 6.5 **(a, b)** Chronic duodenal ulcer. Ulcer with a clean base present on the anterior wall. Note the deformed bulb and the pseudodiverticula.

Endoscopic features of chronic duodenal ulcer

- Deformity
- Scarring
- Pseudodiverticulum (outpouching of the mucosa)
- Luminal narrowing

Giant duodenal ulcer is defined as an ulcer with a diameter of more than 2 cm.

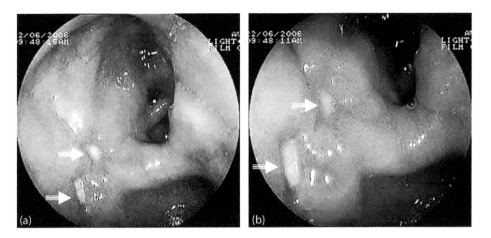

Figure 6.6 **(a, b)** Deformed duodenal bulb, ulcers (arrows) on the anterior wall and pseudodiverticula.

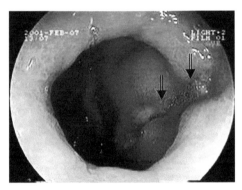

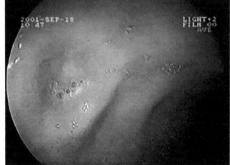

Figure 6.7 Ulcer (arrows) extending across the pylorus into the posterior wall of duodenum.

Figure 6.8 A healing ulcer on the anterior wall of D1.

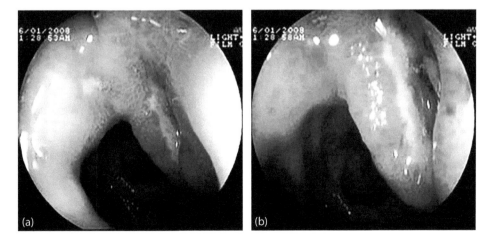

Figure 6.9 **(a, b)** Ulcer on the posterior wall extending from the pylorus.

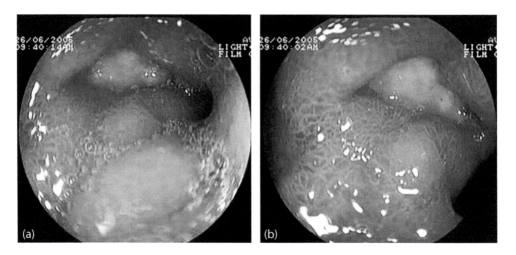

Figure 6.10 (a, b) A deep ulcer on the anterior wall of D1.

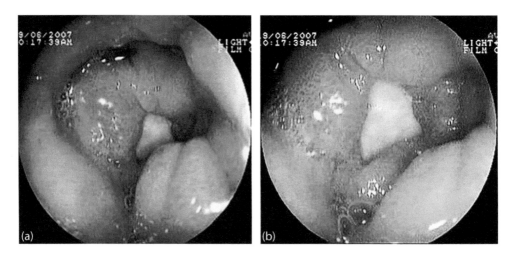

Figure 6.11 (a, b) Deformed duodenal bulb and an active ulcer on the anterior wall.

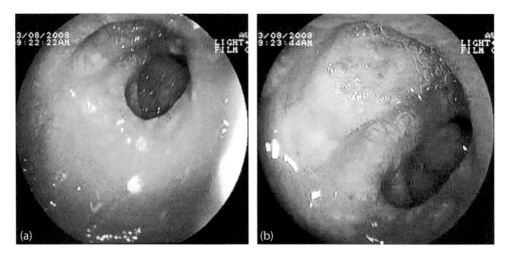

Figure 6.12 (a, b) A giant ulcer on the anterior wall of D1.

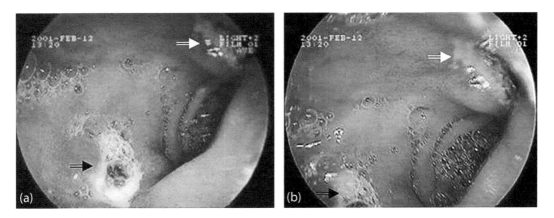

Figure 6.13 (a, b) "Kissing ulcers" on the superior (white arrow) and inferior wall (black arrow) in D1.

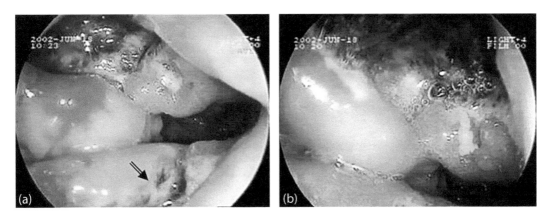

Figure 6.14 (a, b) Giant "kissing ulcers" in D1. Note the ulcer on the inferior wall (arrow).

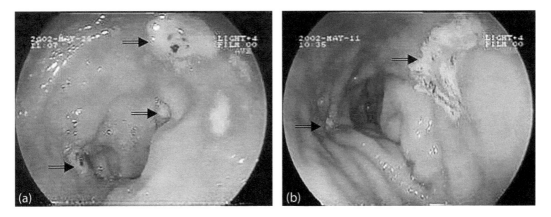

Figure 6.15 (a, b) Multiple ulcers (arrows) in D1.

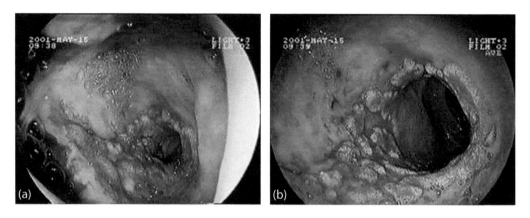

Figure 6.16 **(a, b)** Duodenal bulb showing extensive ulceration and Brunner's gland hyperplasia.

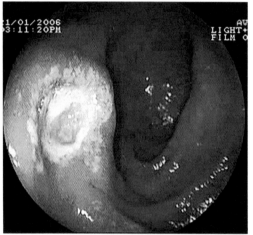

Figure 6.17 Ulcer with surrounding edema in D1.

Figure 6.18 Multiple superficial ulcers in D2.

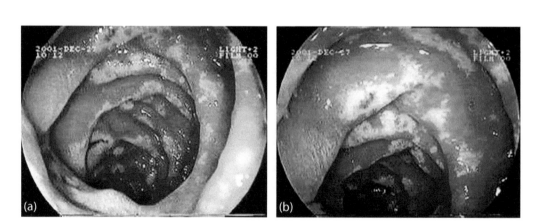

Figure 6.19 **(a, b)** Multiple erosions involving D2.

Complications of duodenal ulcer
- Acute
  - Bleeding
  - Perforation
- Chronic
  - Gastric outlet obstruction
  - Bilioduodenal fistula/bile duct stricture

Endoscopic stigmata of ulcer bleeding
- High risk
  - Spurting pulsatile bleeding
  - Oozing ulcer base
  - Visible vessel
  - Adherent clot
- Low risk
  - Flat pigmented/red spot
  - Clean ulcer base

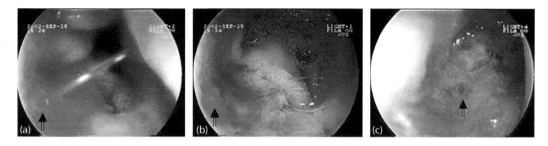

Figure 6.20 **(a)** Spurting bleeding from the ulcer base (arrow) in D1. **(b)** Bleeding was controlled by injecting adrenaline and saline into the ulcer base. **(c)** Visible vessel (arrow) in the ulcer base as seen 48 h later.

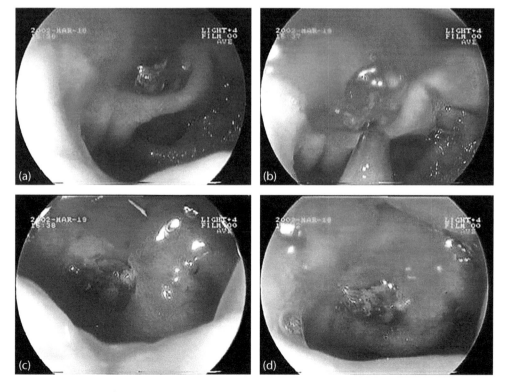

Figure 6.21 **(a)** Actively oozing ulcer in D1. **(b)** The ulcer base was injected with adrenaline:saline 1: 10,000. **(c, d)** Ulcer base as seen after endoscopic control of bleeding.

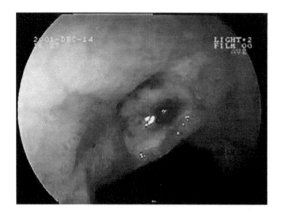

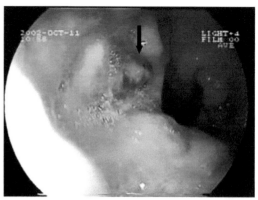

Figure 6.22 "Visible vessel" in the ulcer base.

Figure 6.23 Ulcer and the "visible vessel" (arrow).

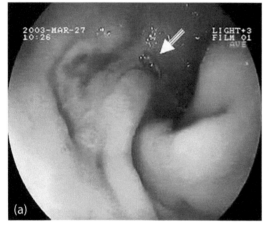

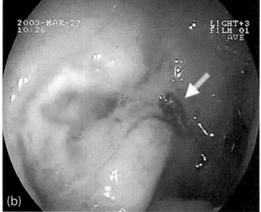

Figure 6.24 (a, b) "Visible vessel" (arrow) in an otherwise clean ulcer base.

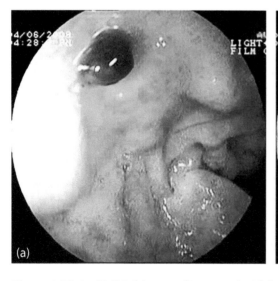

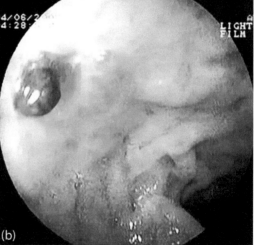

Figure 6.25 (a, b) "Visible vessel" covered with fresh clot.

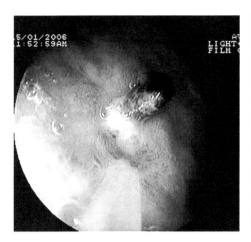

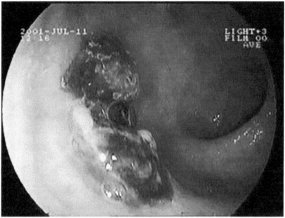

Figure 6.26 "Visible vessel" accentuated by adherent clot.

Figure 6.27 Ulcer on the anterior wall covered with clot.

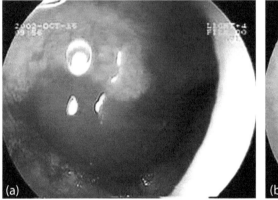

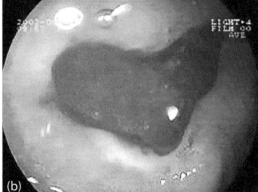

Figure 6.28 (a, b) Ulcer on the anterior wall completely covered with a fresh clot.

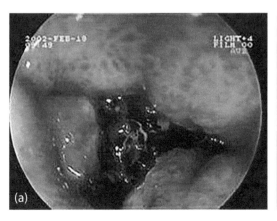

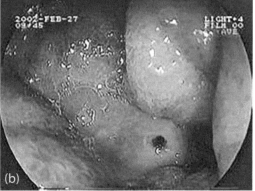

Figure 6.29 (a) A deep ulcer partially covered with clot. (b) Same ulcer eight days later. The clot has been replaced by a "flat red spot."

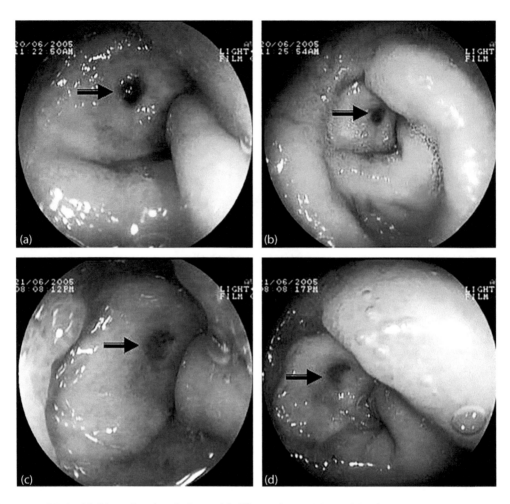

Figure 6.30 **(a, b)** Giant duodenal ulcer with "flat red spot" (arrow) in the center. **(c, d)** Appearance 24 h later.

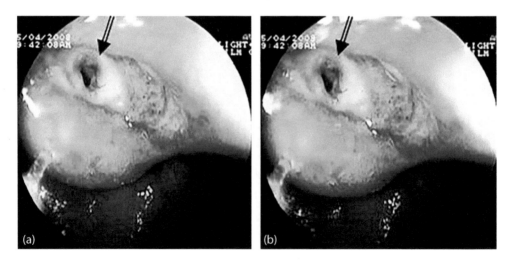

Figure 6.31 **(a–b)** Ulcer on the antero-superior wall of D1 showing a perforation (arrow) in the center. *(Continued)*

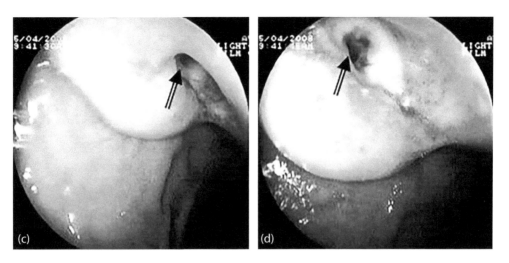

Figure 6.31 (Continued) **(c–d)** Ulcer on the antero-superior wall of D1 showing a perforation (arrow) in the center.

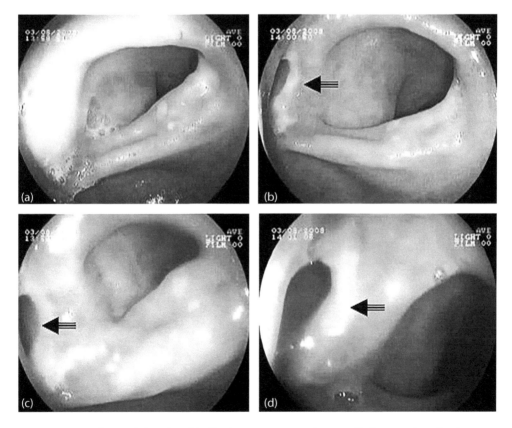

Figure 6.32 **(a)** Deformed duodenal bulb showing accumulation of bilio-purulent fluid. **(b–d)** A perforated ulcer (arrow) was seen lying below the fluid.

Suspected perforation is an absolute contraindication for endoscopy. In both of the above cases, clinical signs and symptoms were misleading, suggesting acute exacerbation of duodenal ulcer only.

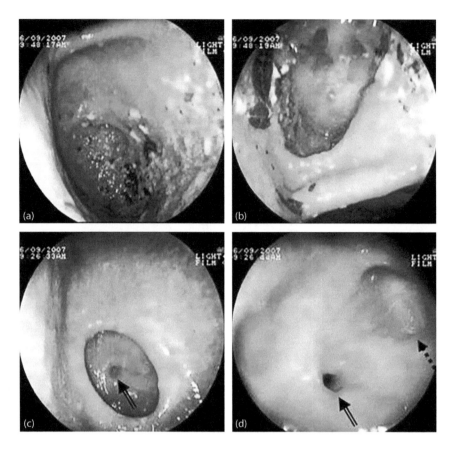

Figure 6.33 Duodenal stenosis: **(a)** Food residue in the antrum and **(b)** fundus. **(c)** Deformed duodenal bulb and the pinhole opening (arrow) seen through pylorus. **(d)** Duodenal bulb. Note the pseudodiverticulum (broken arrow) and the pinhole opening (arrow) at its center.

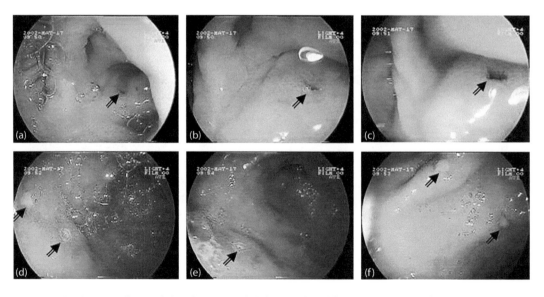

Figure 6.34 **(a–c)** Deformed duodenum with bilioduodenal fistula (arrow). **(d–f)** Multiple superficial ulcers (arrow) in the gastric antrum in the same patient. Possibly, the fistula was secondary to duodenal ulcer penetration. Though no active ulcer was noted in D1, the deformed duodenum indicated its earlier existence.

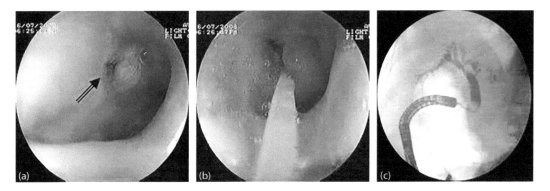

Figure 6.35 (a) Choledochoduodenal fistula. Bile was seen pooling in D1 through a tiny opening at the (arrow) apex. (b) Cannulation and injection of contrast opacified the common bile duct. (c) Opacification of proximal biliary tree confirms presence of bilioduodenal fistula. Distal biliary tree did not opacify because of stricture at the fistula site.

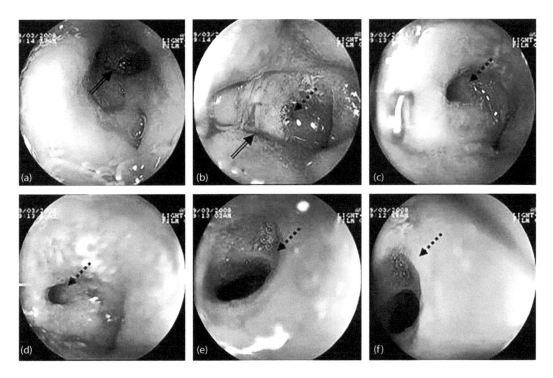

Figure 6.36 Choledochoduodenal fistula. (a) Deformed D1. An ulcer (arrow) was seen on the superior wall. (b) Close-up view of the ulcer (arrow) revealed a tiny opening (broken arrow) in its base exuding bile. (c–f) Further inspection of the opening (broken arrow) confirmed it to be the bile duct.

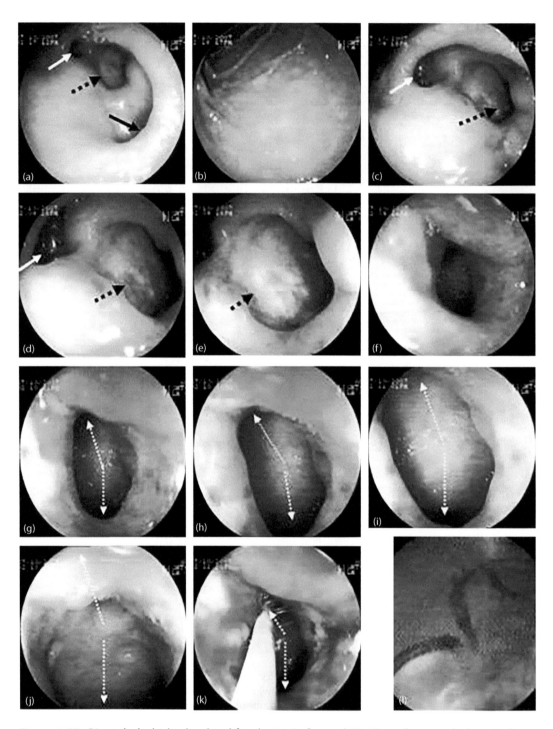

Figure 6.37 Giant choledochoduodenal fistula. (a) Deformed D1. Note the pseudodiverticulum (white arrow), an ulcer (broken arrow) and the passage (arrow) to D2. (b) Normal looking D2. (c–e) Pseudodiverticulum (arrow) and closer view of the ulcer (broken arrow). (f) Probing the medial wall of the ulcer led to an oblong opening. (g–i) Close-up view of the opening suggested it to be a part of the bile duct wall having superior and inferior ends (broken white arrows). (j) The bile duct mucosa was quite distinct in its appearance. (k) The superior opening of the bile duct was cannulated and contrast injected. (l) This opacified the proximal biliary tree, confirming the presence of a large choledochoduodenal fistula.

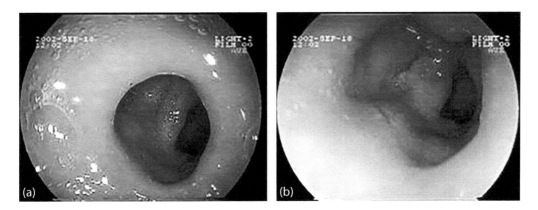

Figure 6.38 (a, b) Deformed D1 with pseudodiverticula following healed duodenal ulcer.

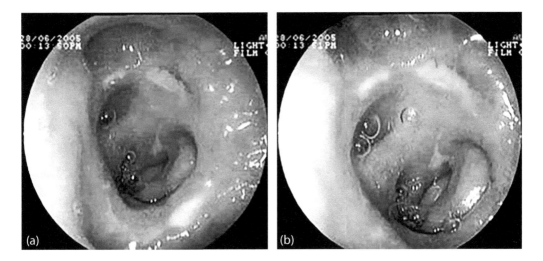

Figure 6.39 (a, b) Deformed D1 with pseudodiverticula and superficial ulcers.

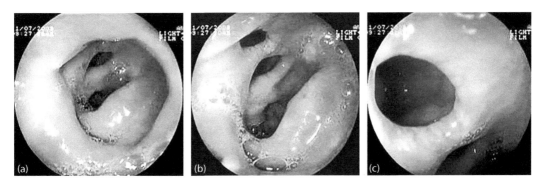

Figure 6.40 (a) Deformed D1 and pseudodiverticuli seen through the pylorus. (b) Closer view of the D1. (c) Close-up view of one of the diverticuli.

7

Gastrojejunostomy

Peptic ulcer surgery accounted for the majority of the cases of gastrojejunostomy (GJ) in the past. With the sharp decline in the incidence of elective surgery for peptic ulcer, the major indication for GJ in the present time is gastric outlet obstruction and partial gastrectomy for various causes. Both early as well late complications of GJ are best evaluated by endoscopy. It is imperative to enter and inspect both the afferent as well as the efferent loop for any pathology.

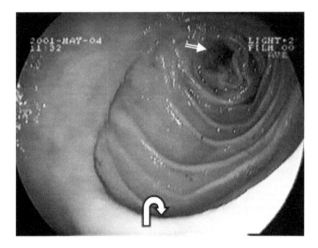

Figure 7.1 Normal gastrojejunostomy (GJ) stoma. The efferent loop opening is clearly seen (straight arrow). The afferent loop opening is hidden below the gastric mucosa (curved arrow).

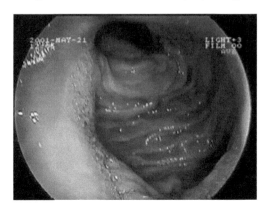

Figure 7.2 GJ stoma.

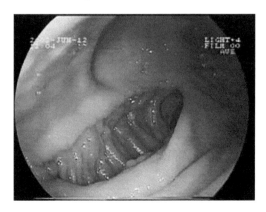

Figure 7.3 GJ stoma along the greater curvature.

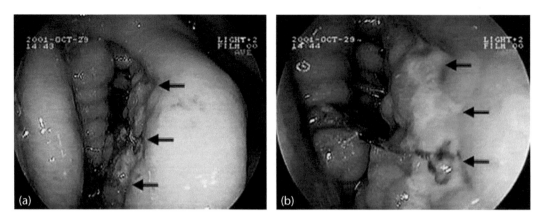

Figure 7.4 **(a, b)** GJ stomal edema. Note the silk suture and the ulceration along the suture line.

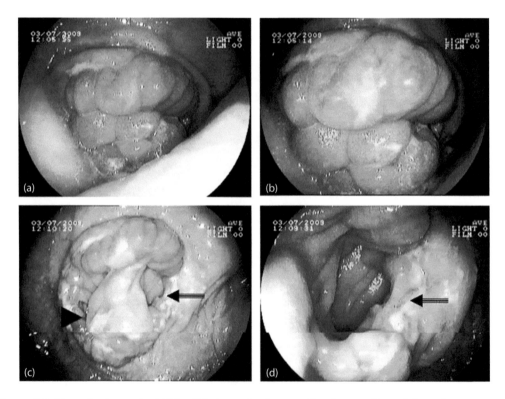

Figure 7.5 Stomal edema. **(a, b)** The GJ stoma is obscured by the two lips of the edematous jejunal mucosa. **(c)** The afferent loop (arrow head) and the efferent loop (arrow) openings were identified by gentle manipulation. **(d)** Close-up view of the efferent loop opening.

Endoscopy in the early postoperative period is fraught with the risk of suture line dehiscence. This is can be minimized by adhering to the following principles:

- Should be performed by an experienced endoscopist only.
- Use minimal distention and force.
- Proceed only if lumen is visible.
- Avoid entering too much into afferent or efferent loops.

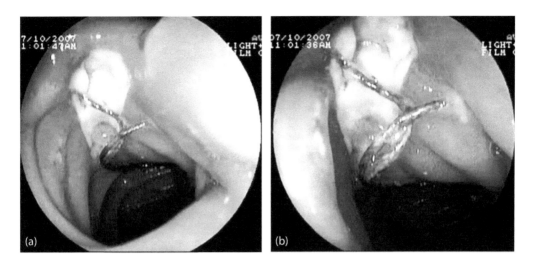

Figure 7.6 (a, b) Stomal ulcer around a silk suture.

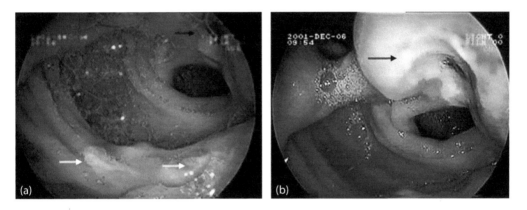

Figure 7.7 (a, b) Stomal ulcer close to efferent loop opening (black arrow). Multiple erosions involving jejunal mucosa (white arrows).

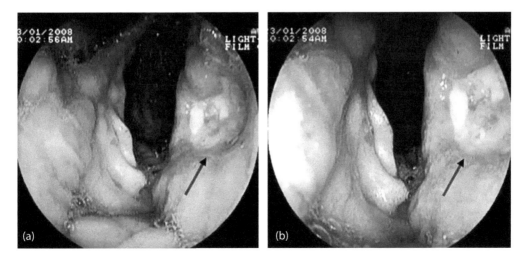

Figure 7.8 (a, b) Giant stomal ulcer (arrow).

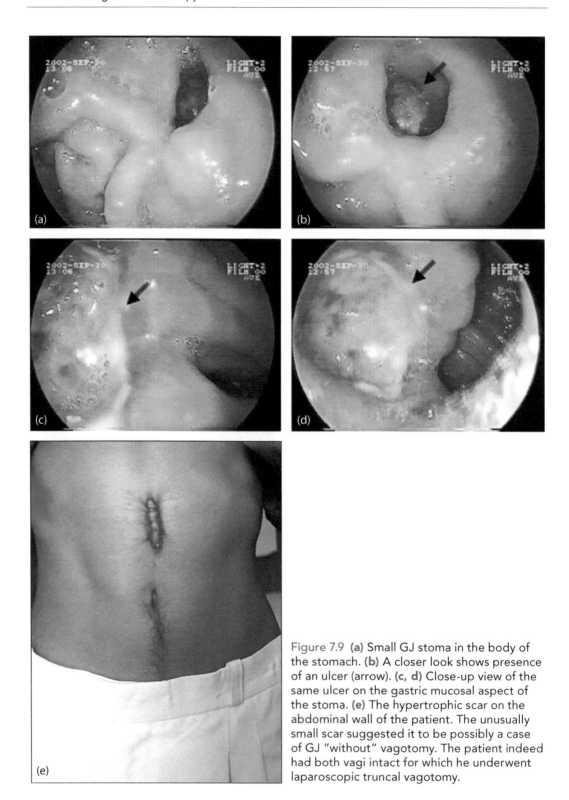

Figure 7.9 (a) Small GJ stoma in the body of the stomach. (b) A closer look shows presence of an ulcer (arrow). (c, d) Close-up view of the same ulcer on the gastric mucosal aspect of the stoma. (e) The hypertrophic scar on the abdominal wall of the patient. The unusually small scar suggested it to be possibly a case of GJ "without" vagotomy. The patient indeed had both vagi intact for which he underwent laparoscopic truncal vagotomy.

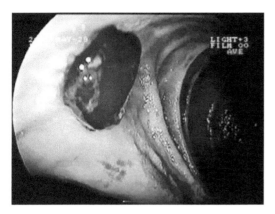

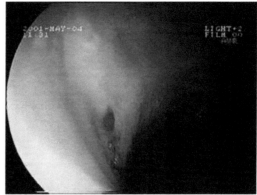

Figure 7.10 GJ stomal ulcer bleeding. A fresh clot covering the ulcer.

Figure 7.11 Stomal ulcer bleeding. "Flat red spot" on the ulcer surface suggested recent hemorrhage.

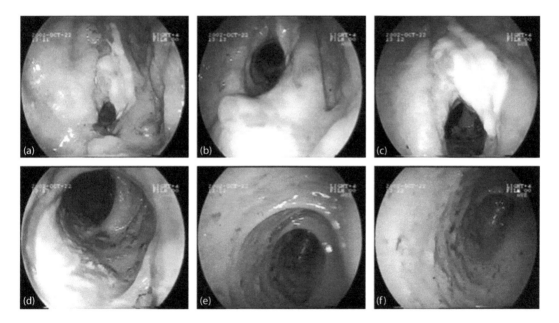

Figure 7.12 (a–f) Gastrojejunocolic fistula. Note the grossly ulcerated stoma and the feculent contents of the efferent loop.

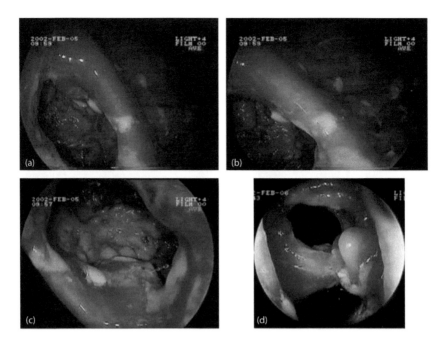

Figure 7.13 Gastrojejunocolic fistula. **(a–c)** Fistulous opening by the side of the GJ stoma containing fecal matter. **(d)** Colonoscopy in the same patient showing two openings in the transverse colon. The lower one was communicating with the stomach. Note staining of the fistulous tract with methylene blue that the patient was made to drink during colonoscopy to confirm the communication.

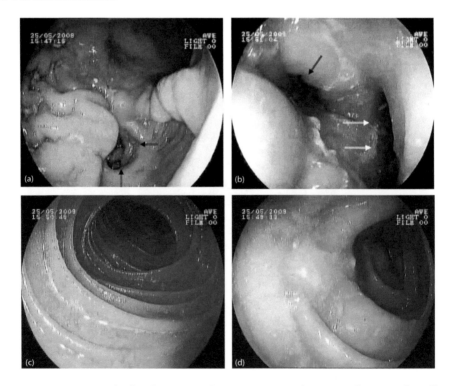

Figure 7.14 Gastrojejunocolic fistula. **(a)** Feculent contents in the stomach. Note the efferent loop opening (arrow). **(b)** A close-up view of the efferent loop opening shows two passages. **(c)** Entry through one of them (white arrows) led to the jejunal lumen. **(d)** Entry through the other one (black arrow) revealed triangular mucosal folds and fecal matter, suggesting colonic lumen, thus confirming presence of gastrojejunocolic fistula.

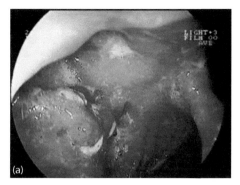

Endoscopic diagnosis of gastrojejunocolic fistula is made on the following findings:

- Feculent contents in the gastric lumen.
- Grossly ulcerated stoma.
- Visualization of colon while manipulating the endoscope through the openings in the stoma.
- Manipulation of the colonoscope in the transverse colon may bring into view jejunal or gastric lumen.
- Chromocolonoscopy: With the colonoscope in the transverse colon, the patient is asked to drink methylene blue dye. Prompt appearance of the dye in the colon confirms presence of a fistula between the stomach and the colon.

Tropical Gastroenterology 2001: 22; 221

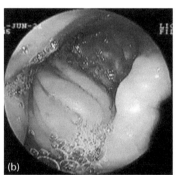
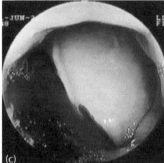
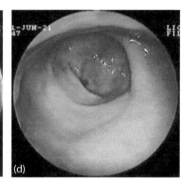

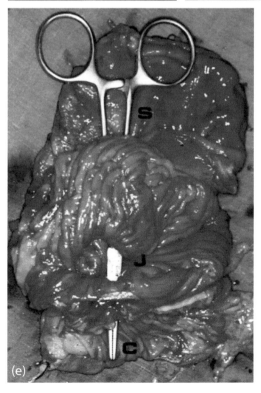

Figure 7.15 Gastrojejunocolic fistula.
(a) Unhealthy GJ stoma with feculent contents. Colonoscopy was performed in the same patient. (b) Jejunal mucosa was visualized as the colonoscope was manipulated in the transverse colon. (c) Gastric mucosa was seen next. This was confirmed by asking the patient to drink methylene blue, which was seen pooling in the stomach. (d) Pylorus was also visualized during the same study. (e) Specimen after *en block* resection, showing stomach (S), jejunal (J), colonic (C) segments and the fistulous communication, marked by the artery forceps.

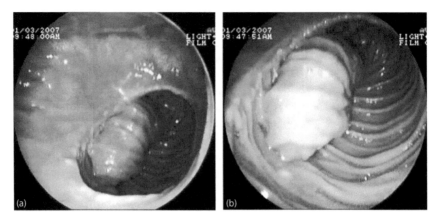

Figure 7.16 (a, b) Retrograde jejunogastric intussusception. This was an incidental finding in a patient who underwent endoscopy for dyspeptic symptoms.

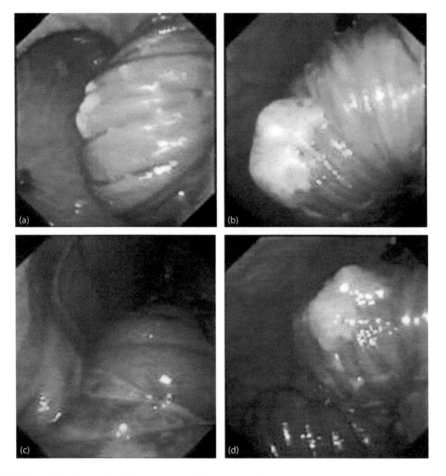

Figure 7.17 (a–d) Retrograde jejunogastric intussusception.

Retrograde jejunogastric intussusception is a relatively uncommon complication of gastrojejunostomy. Efferent loop intussusception is more frequent than afferent loop. The usual presenting features are pain, coffee-ground vomiting and an ill-defined lump in the epigastrium. Diagnosis is confirmed on endoscopy. Early surgery is indicated to prevent strangulation of the jejunal segment.

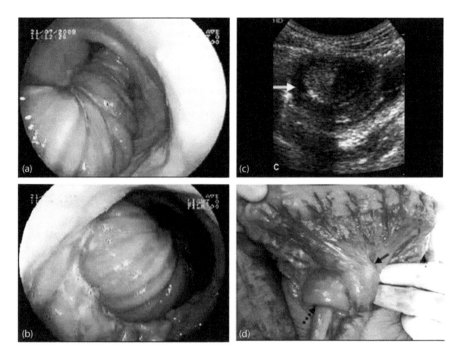

Figure 7.18 **(a–b)** Retrograde jejunogastric intussusception. **(c)** Abdominal ultrasonography showing a circular hyperechoic mass (arrow) inside stomach – the "'target sign." **(d)** Operative photograph showing transmesocolic afferent loop (arrow) and the intussuscepted efferent loop (broken arrow).

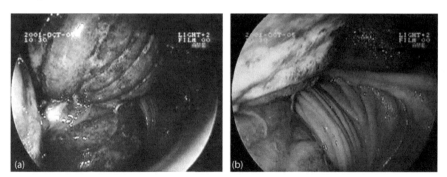

Figure 7.19 **(a, b)** Retrograde jejunogastric intussusception. Jejunal loop congested and pregangrenous.

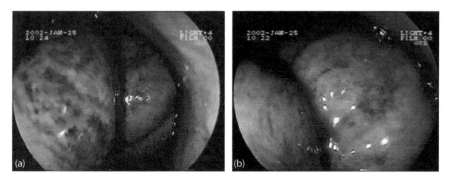

Figure 7.20 **(a, b)** Retrograde jejunogastric intussusception. Note the gangrenous jejunal loop.

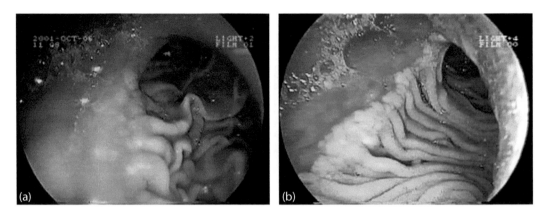

Figure 7.21 (a, b) Bile reflux gastritis. Note the sharply demarcated gastric mucosa because of the inflammation.

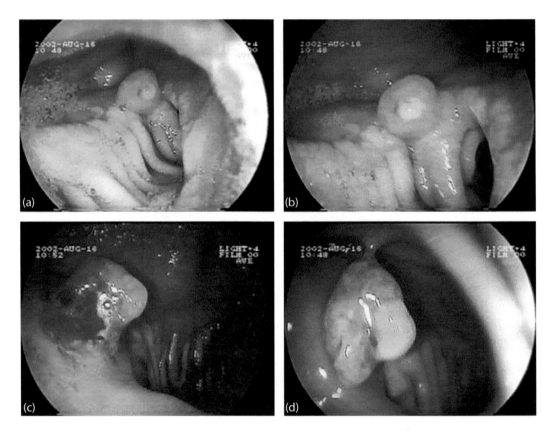

Figure 7.22 (a, b) Inflammatory polyp close to the efferent loop opening in a patient with severe bile reflux gastritis. (c, d) Another polyp close to the afferent loop opening. The patient presented with recurrent anemia.

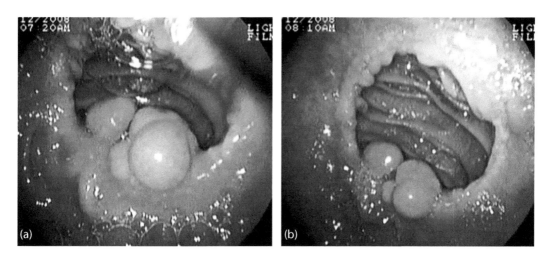

Figure 7.23 (a, b) Inflammatory polyps at the GJ stomal margin.

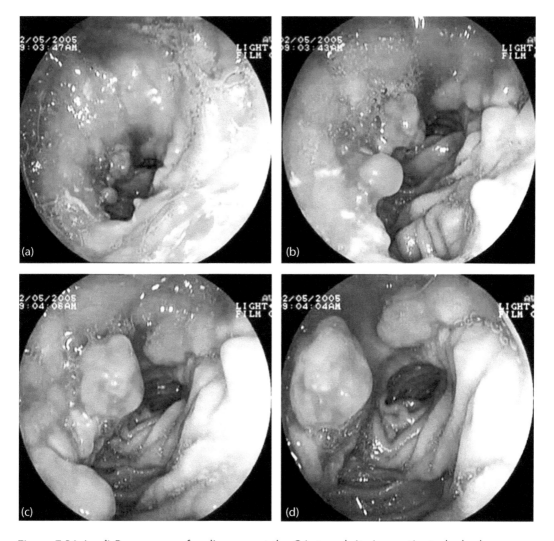

Figure 7.24 (a–d) Recurrence of malignancy at the GJ stomal site in a patient who had undergone subtotal gastrectomy for carcinoma two years back.

8

Benign tumors

Gastrointestinal stromal tumor (GIST) is the commonest non-epithelial tumor of the GI tract. It arises from the interstitial cells of Cajal, a part of the autonomic nervous system located in the muscular propria. The stomach is the commonest site of its occurrence, followed by the small bowel, the esophagus and the colorectum. It commonly presents with bleeding. Mucosal biopsy is usually non-yielding; deeper biopsy may be required for diagnosis. The presence of spindle cells points to the diagnosis of GIST that is further confirmed on positive immunohistology for CD 117 (*c-kit*). Surgical excision is the preferred treatment. Tumor size <2 cm and a mitotic index <5/50 HPF suggest a low risk tumor.

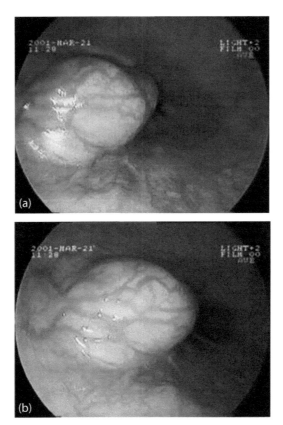

Figure 8.1 **(a, b)** GIST at the lower end of the esophagus. This was an incidental finding on endoscopy for dyspepsia.

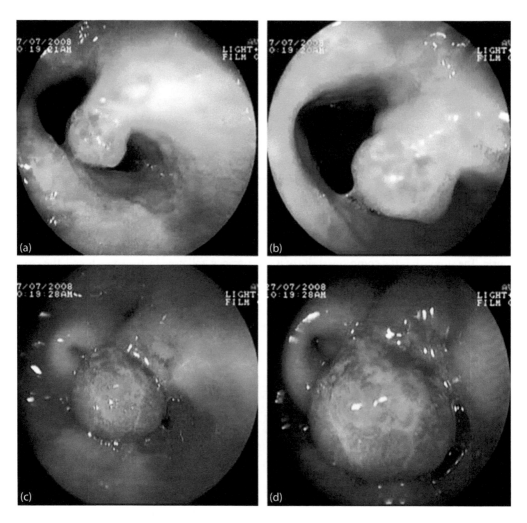

Figure 8.2 **(a–d)** Sentinel polyp. Inflammatory polyp at the GE junction. This is more often an incidental finding on endoscopy.

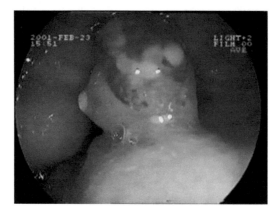

Figure 8.3 Inflammatory polyp at the GE junction.

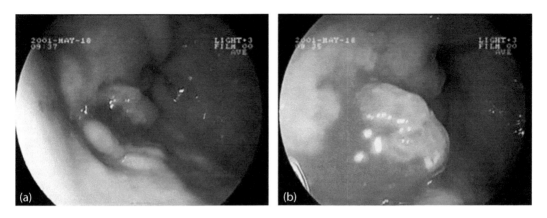

Figure 8.4 (**a, b**) Bleeding inflammatory polyp at the GE junction.

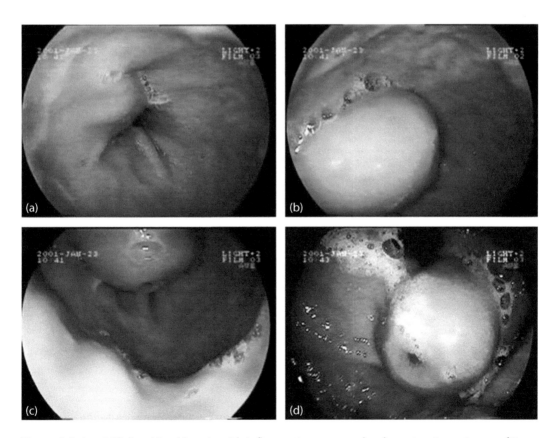

Figure 8.5 (**a–c**) Sliding hiatal hernia with inflammatory mucosal polyp, at various stages of its appearance during endoscopy. (**d**) The same polyp, prolapsing below the GE junction, was seen on retroflexion. Note the central ulceration.

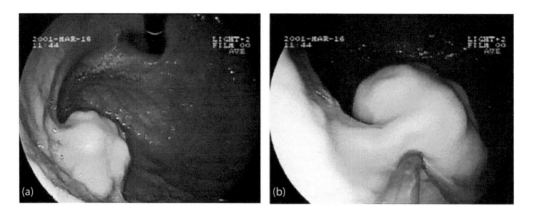

Figure 8.6 (a, b) GIST in the gastric fundus.

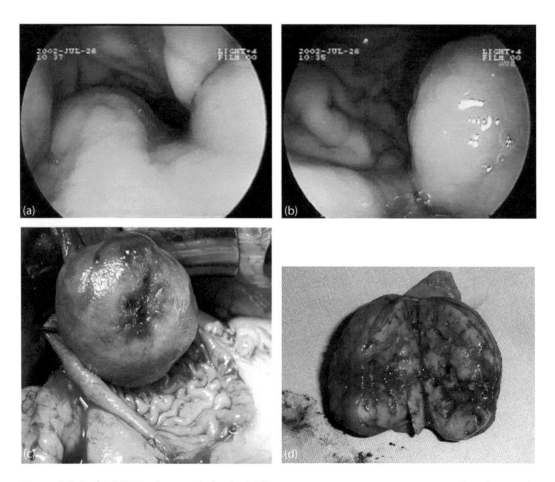

Figure 8.7 (a, b) GIST in the gastric body. (c) Tumor as seen on gastrotomy. Note the ulcerated center, the site of bleeding in this patient. (d) Bisected tumor after excision.

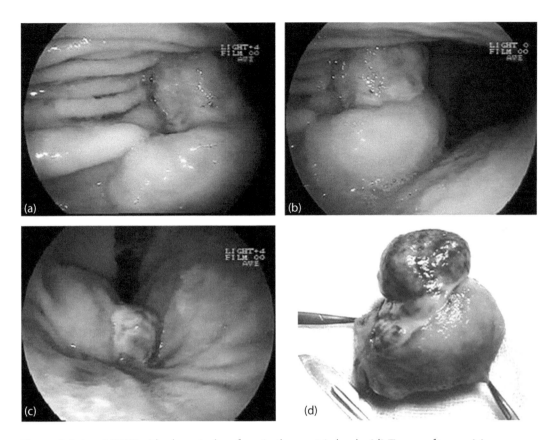

Figure 8.8 (a–c) GIST with ulcerated surface in the gastric body. (d) Tumor after excision.

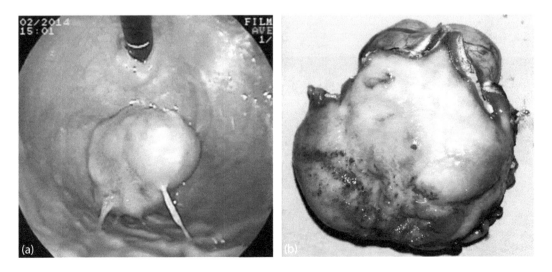

Figure 8.9 (a) GIST in the gastric fundus. (b) Tumor after excision.

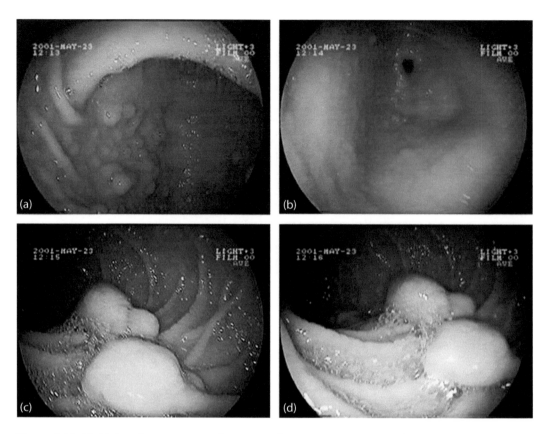

Figure 8.10 Multiple adenomatous polyps in (a) the gastric antrum, (b) the prepyloric region and (c, d) D2

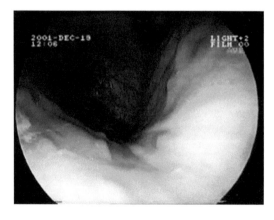

Figure 8.11 Multiple inflammatory polyps in the fundus.

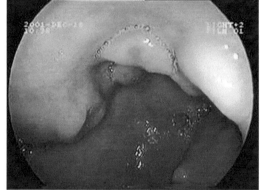

Figure 8.12 Inflammatory polyps in the antrum.

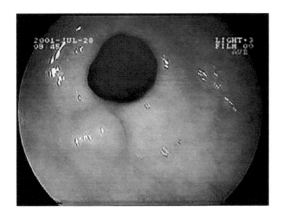

Figure 8.13 Prepyloric submucosal polyp.

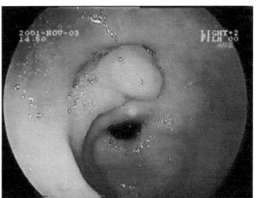

Figure 8.14 Prepyloric inflammatory polyp.

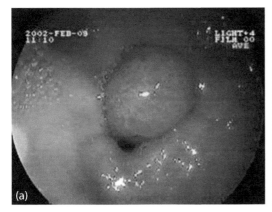

Figure 8.15 (a, b) Inflammatory polyp obstructing pylorus.

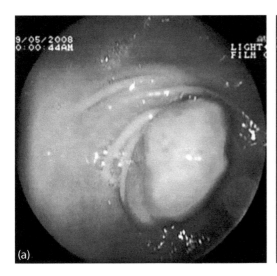
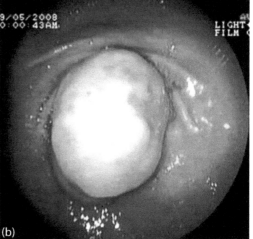

Figure 8.16 (a, b) An inflammatory polyp arising from the pyloric ring. The patient presented with recurrent hematemesis and melena.

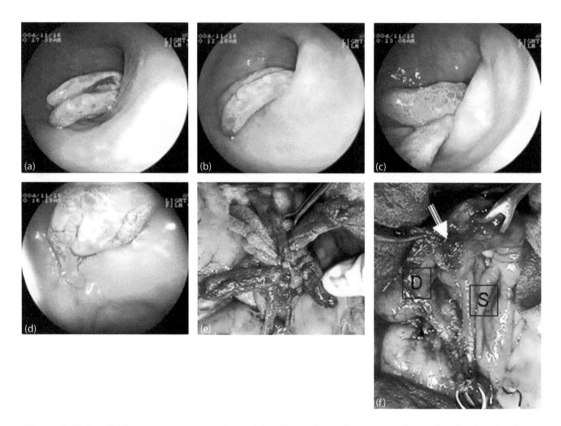

Figure 8.17 (a–d) Hamartomatous polyp arising from the pyloric ring. The polyp had multiple finger-like projections converging on a single stalk. (e) The polyp during surgical excision. (f) The stalk (arrow) after excision. The polyp was an incidental detection in an elderly man who underwent endoscopy for dyspepsia.

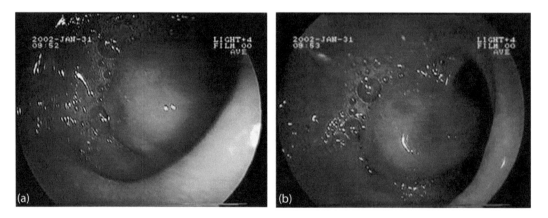

Figure 8.18 (a, b) GIST at the junction of D1 and D2.The patient presented with recurrent melena.

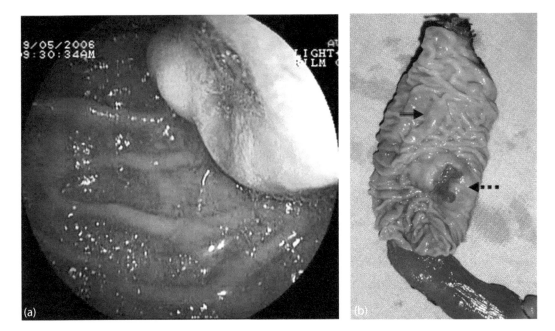

Figure 8.19 **(a)** GIST in the second part of the duodenum. **(b)** Pancreaticoduodenectomy specimen showing the ulcerated tumor (broken arrow). Note the position of ampulla of Vater (arrow). The patient, a middle-aged man, presented with recurrent episodes of melena.

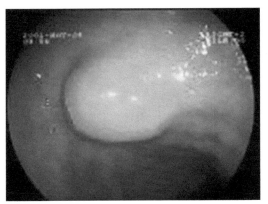

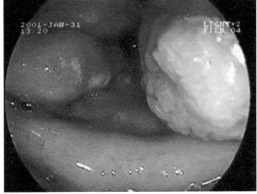

Figure 8.20 Submucosal lipoma at the apex of D1.

Figure 8.21 Villous adenoma in D2.

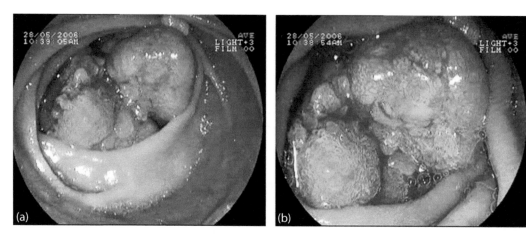

Figure 8.22 **(a, b)** Villous adenoma completely filling the D2 lumen. The patient, a middle-aged woman, presented with anemia and retention vomiting.

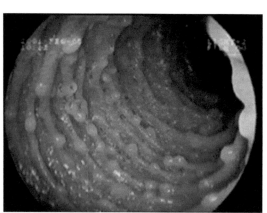

Figure 8.23 Lymphoid hyperplasia in D2.

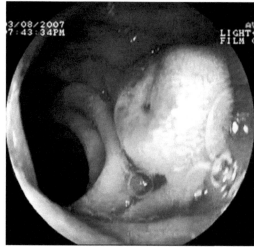

Figure 8.24 Ulcerated stalk in D2.The patient presented with bleeding 10 days after snare polypectomy.

9

Malignant tumors

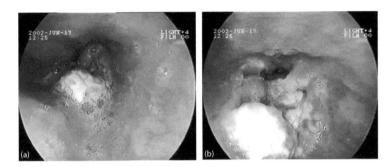

Figure 9.1 **(a, b)** Ulcero-proliferative squamous cell carcinoma in the mid-esophagus.

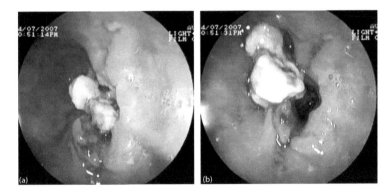

Figure 9.2 **(a, b)** Squamous cell carcinoma in the mid-esophagus. Note the impacted food debris (whitish material).

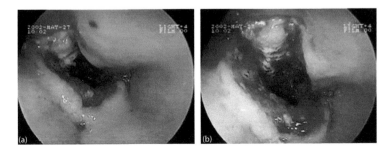

Figure 9.3 **(a, b)** Squamous cell carcinoma, ulcerated tumor.

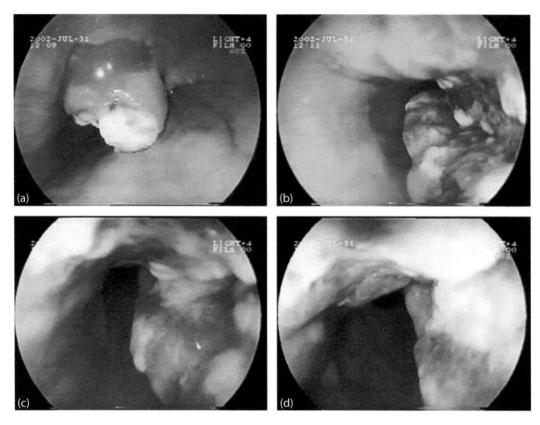

Figure 9.4 (a–d) Squamous cell carcinoma in the mid-esophagus.

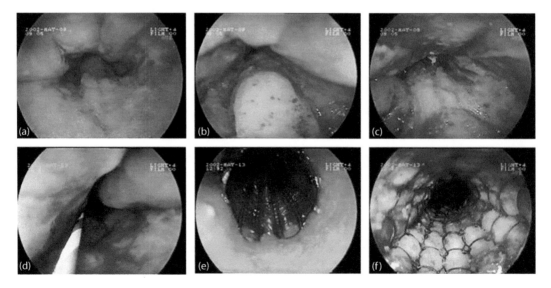

Figure 9.5 (a–c) Squamous cell carcinoma involving the mid-esophagus. (d) Distal tumor-free lumen with guidewire in place. (e, f) Self-expandable metal prosthesis across the tumor.

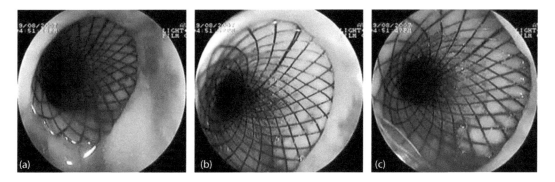

Figure 9.6 **(a–c)** Self-expendable metal stent across an inoperable tumor in the mid-esophagus.

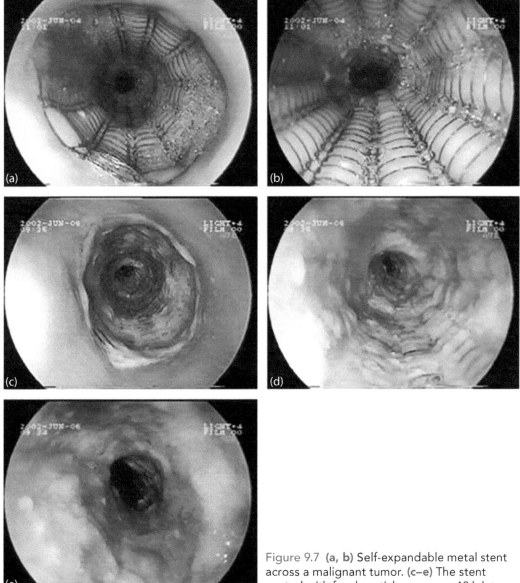

Figure 9.7 **(a, b)** Self-expandable metal stent across a malignant tumor. **(c–e)** The stent coated with food particles, as seen 48 h later.

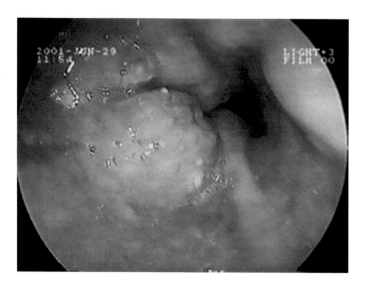

Figure 9.8 Early carcinoma in the distal esophagus.

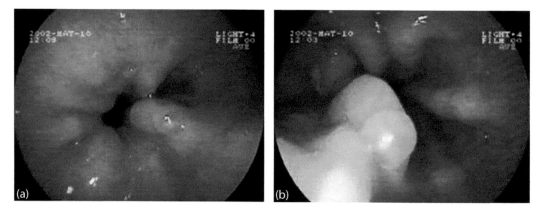

Figure 9.9 (a, b) Small polyp at the Z line. Clinically, the polyp was thought to be inflammatory (sentinel polyp); biopsy revealed in situ carcinoma.

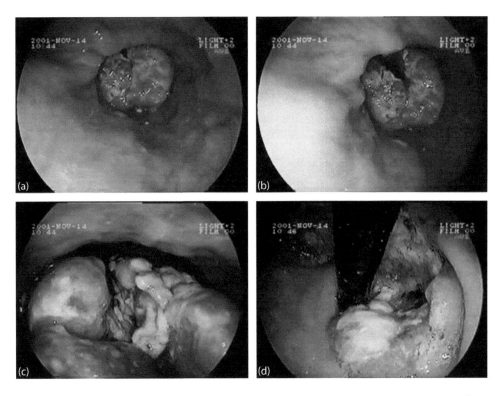

Figure 9.10 (a–c) Adenocarcinoma at the lower end of the esophagus. (d) View on retroflexion showing extension of the tumor into the stomach.

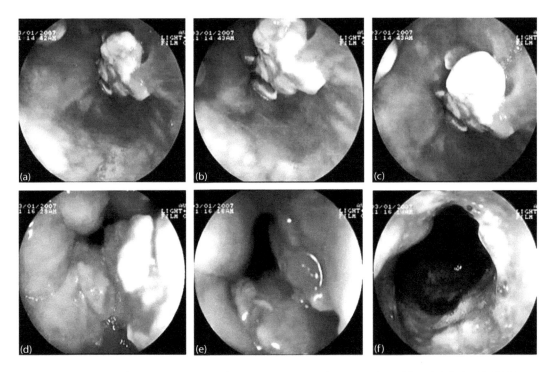

Figure 9.11 (a–c) Adenocarcinoma at the GE junction with accumulated food debris. (d–f) View after removal of the food debris. Increased circumferential involvement distally.

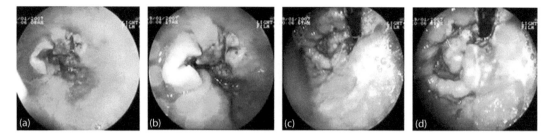

Figure 9.12 **(a, b)** Adenocarcinoma at the GE junction. **(c, d)** View on retroflexion.

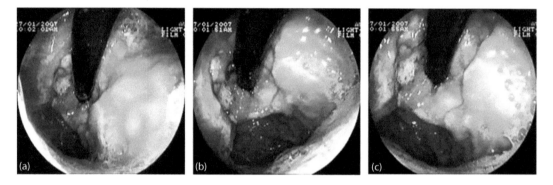

Figure 9.13 **(a–c)** Ulcerated tumor at the GE junction; view on retroflexion.

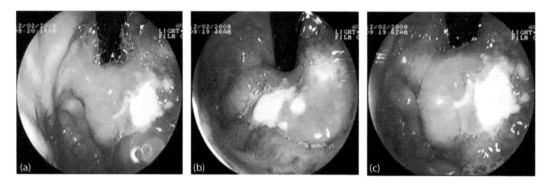

Figure 9.14 **(a–c)** Adenocarcinoma at the GE junction. The tumor extension into the stomach as seen on retroflexion.

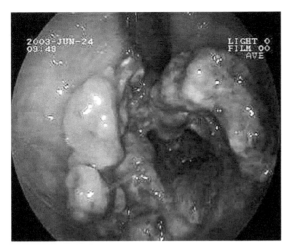

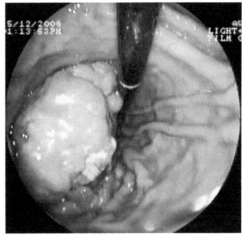

Figure 9.15 Ulcerated tumor involving the gastric fundus.

Figure 9.16 Polypoidal tumor filling the entire fundus.

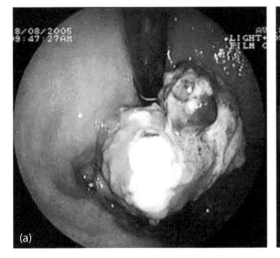

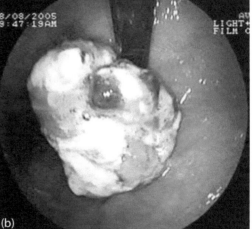

(a)

(b)

Figure 9.17 (a, b) Polypoidal adenocarcinoma below the GE junction.

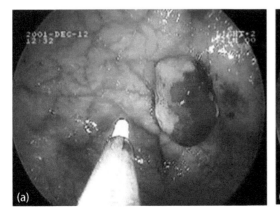

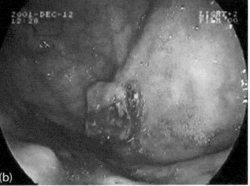

(a)

(b)

Figure 9.18 (a, b) Bleeding polypoidal tumor in the fundus.

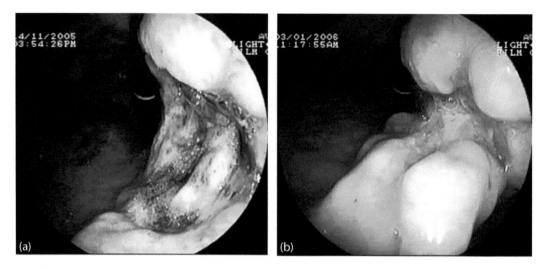

Figure 9.19 **(a)** Giant ulcer with necrotic base involving lesser curve. Endoscopic biopsy was negative for malignancy; hence the patient was treated with proton pump inhibitors alone. **(b)** Partial healing was apparent on repeat endoscopy about six weeks later. But the biopsy from the ulcer margin this time revealed evidence of carcinoma.

Malignant ulcers may also show signs of healing on conservative management. Strict follow-up to demonstrate complete healing and repeated biopsies are mandatory to exclude malignancy.

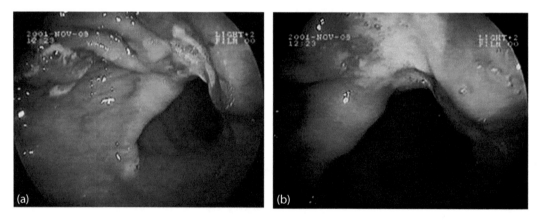

Figure 9.20 **(a, b)** Malignant ulcer involving the lesser curve and incisura.

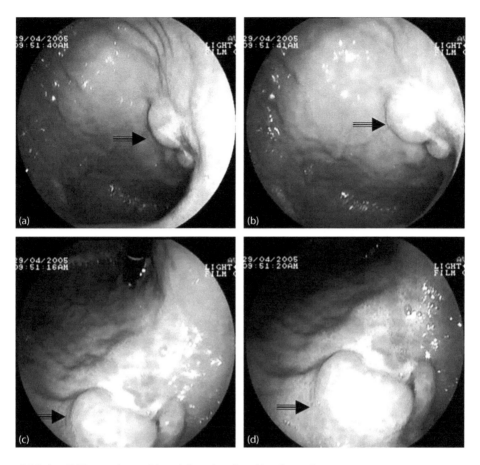

Figure 9.21 (a–d) Tumor (arrow) involving the distal body and antrum.

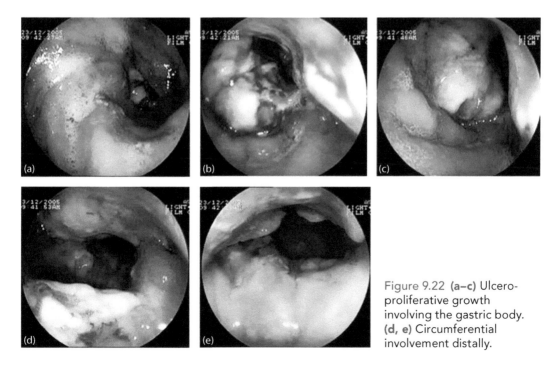

Figure 9.22 (a–c) Ulcero-proliferative growth involving the gastric body. (d, e) Circumferential involvement distally.

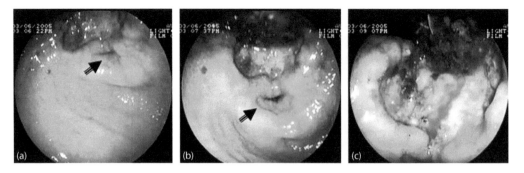

Figure 9.23 **(a–c)** Ulcerated tumor starting from the incisura to the pylorus (arrow).

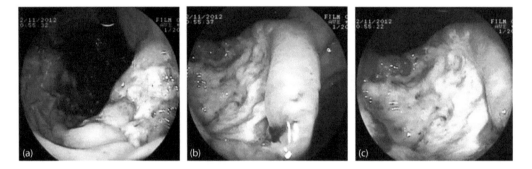

Figure 9.24 **(a–c)** Ulcerated tumor involving the incisura and the lesser curvature. View on retroflexion.

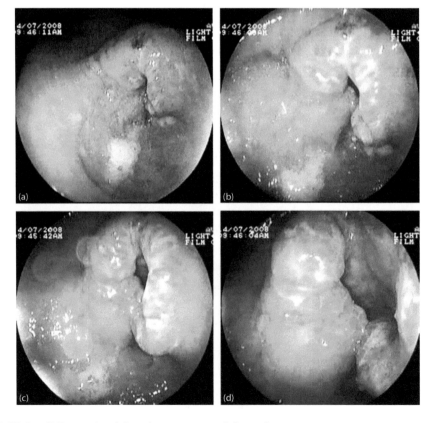

Figure 9.25 **(a–d)** Tumor involving the antrum and the pylorus.

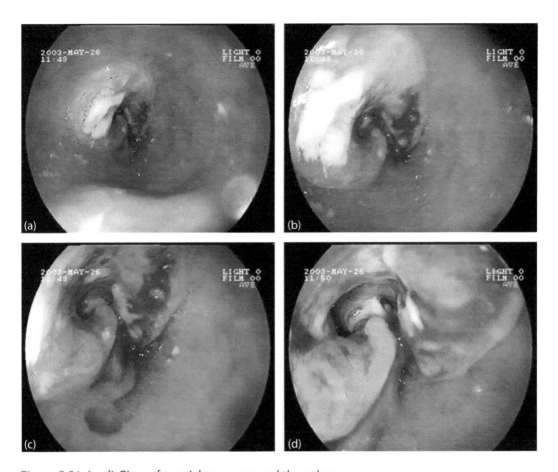

Figure 9.26 **(a–d)** Circumferential tumor around the pylorus.

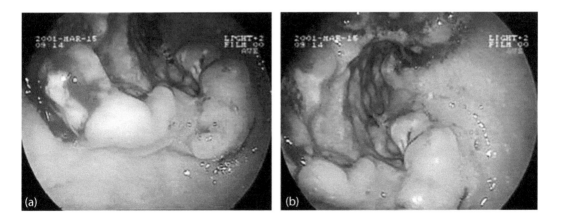

Figure 9.27 **(a, b)** Ulcerated tumor around the pylorus

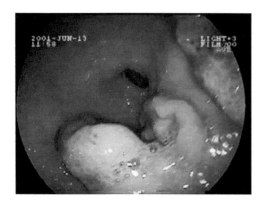

Figure 9.28 Polypoidal tumor in the antrum.

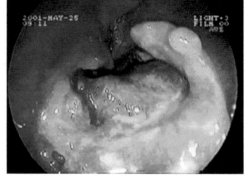

Figure 9.29 Ulcerated tumor around the pylorus.

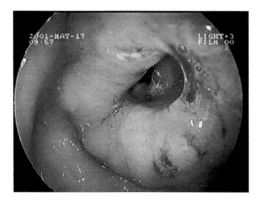

Figure 9.30 Polypoidal tumor around the pylorus.

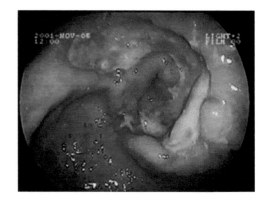

Figure 9.31 Ulcerated tumor with elevated margin around the pylorus.

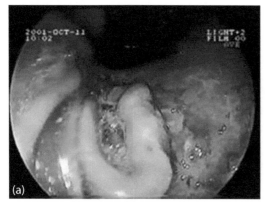

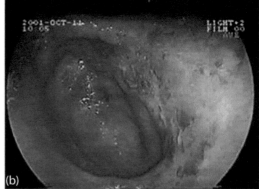

Figure 9.32 (a, b) Superficial spreading carcinoma involving the body and antrum.

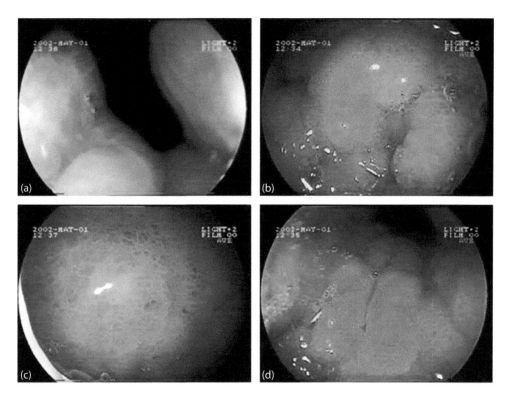

Figure 9.33 (a–d) Linitis plastica; pangastric involvement.

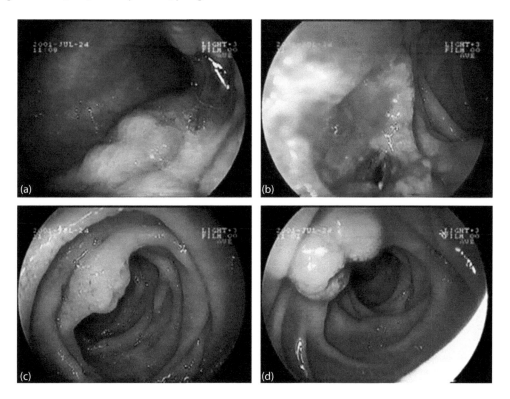

Figure 9.34 (a) Tumor in the gastric antrum extending into (b) the duodenal bulb.
(c, d) Synchronous tumor in the second part of duodenum in the same patient.

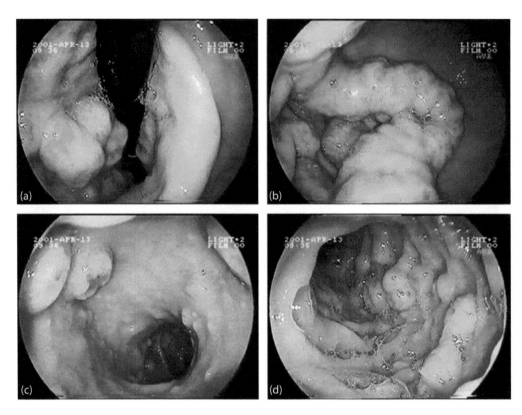

Figure 9.35 Metachronous secondary from a malignant pituitary tumor involving (a, b) the gastric body, (c) the duodenal bulb, (d) D2. The patient, a young man, had undergone excision of prolactinoma four years back.

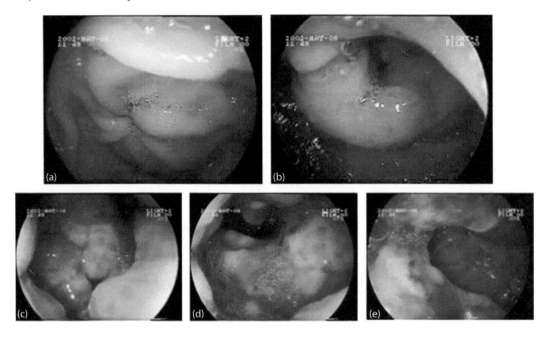

Figure 9.36 Duodenal carcinoma. (a) Normal-appearing pyloric mucosa with evidence of submucosal infiltration. (b) Infiltrated pylorus. (c, d) Tumor involving D1. (e) Tumor abruptly stopping at the junction of D1 and D2.

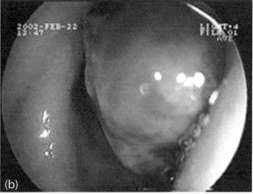
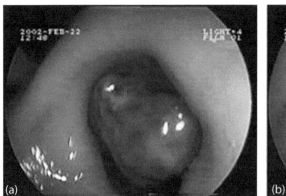

Figure 9.37 (a, b) Polypoidal tumor (adenocarcinoma) in D1. The patient, a 21-year-old man, presented with hematemesis.

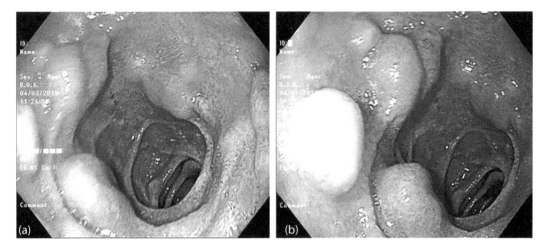

Figure 9.38 (a, b) Multiple submucosal polyps in D1. A deep mucosal biopsy was suggestive of neuroendocrine tumor (NET). The patient, a 52-year-old woman, presented with upper abdominal pain.

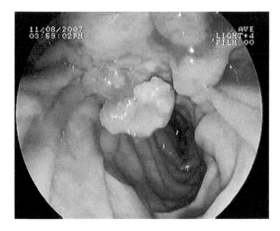

Figure 9.39 Ampullary carcinoma.

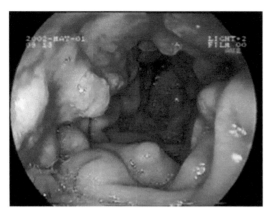

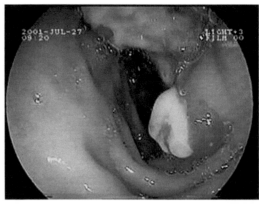

Figure 9.40 Circumferential involvement of D2 secondary to pancreatic head carcinoma.

Figure 9.41 Duodenal infiltration by renal cell carcinoma.

10

Portal hypertension

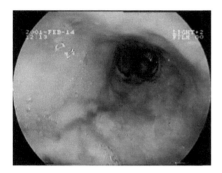

Figure 10.1 Early varices

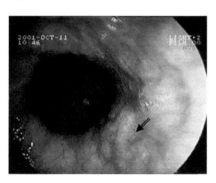

Figure 10.2 Single column early varix (arrow).

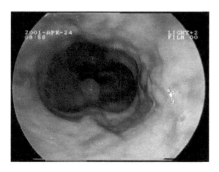

Figure 10.3 Early varices.

CONN'S GRADING

Grade I: Small varices detectable only on performance of Valsalva maneuver.
Grade II: Small varices (diameter of 1–3 mm) visible without Valsalva maneuver.
Grade III: Varices with diameter of 3–6 mm.
Grade IV: Varices > 6 mm in diameter.

MODIFIED DAGRADI GRADING

Grade 1: Blue or red varices <2 mm in diameter.
Grade 2: Blue varices 2–3 mm in diameter.
Grade 3: Elevated blue veins 3–4 mm in diameter.
Grade 4: Tortuous blue varices >4 mm in diameter, almost meeting in the midline.
Grade 5: Grape-like varices occluding the lumen and showing the presence of small cherry-red varices overlying blue-grey varices.

PAQUET'S GRADING

Grade I: Small varices without luminal prolapse.
Grade II: Moderately sized varices showing luminal prolapse with minimal obscuring of the GE junction.
Grade III: Large varices showing luminal prolapse with substantial obscuring of the GE junction.
Grade IV: Very large varices completely obscuring the GE junction.

MODIFIED PAQUET'S GRADING

Grade I: Varices extending just above the mucosal level.
Grade II: Varices projecting by one-third of the luminal diameter that cannot be compressed with air insufflation.
Grade III: Varices projecting up to 50% of the luminal diameter and in contact with each other.

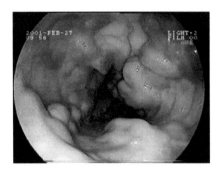

Figure 10.4 Blue varices.

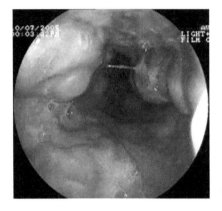

Figure 10.5 Three columns of blue varices.

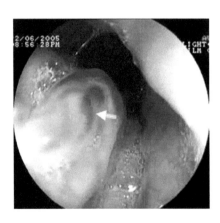

Figure 10.6 "Red wale" mark (arrow) on the varix.

WESTABY'S GRADING

Grade 1: Varices appearing as slight protrusions above mucosa, which can be depressed with insufflations.

Grade 2: Varices occupying <50% of the lumen.

Grade 3: Varices occupying >50% of the lumen and which are very close to each other with confluent appearance.

SOEHENDRA CLASSIFICATION

Grade I: Mild dilatation; diameter <2 mm; barely rising above the relaxed esophagus; more marked in head-down position.

Grade II: Moderate dilatation; tortuous; diameter 3–4 mm; limited to the lower part of the esophagus.

Grade III: Total dilatation; taut; diameter >4 mm; thin-walled; varices upon varices; in the gastric fundus.

Grade IV: Total dilatation; taut; occupy the entire esophagus; frequent presence of gastric or duodenal varices.

ENDOSCOPIC RECORDING OF ESOPHAGEAL VARICES (JAPANESE RESEARCH SOCIETY FOR PORTAL HYPERTENSION)

1. Fundamental color
   a. White (Cw)
   b. Blue (Cb)

2. Red color signs (RCS): (small dilated vessels or micro-telangiectasia on varix surface)
   a. Red wale marking (RWM)
   b. Cherry-red spot (CRS)
   c. Hematocystic spot (HCS)
   d. Diffuse redness (DR)

3. Form
   a. Small, straight varices (F1)
   b. Enlarged tortuous varices occupying <one-third of lumen (F2)
   c. Large coil-shaped varices occupying >one-third of lumen (F3)

4. Location (longitudinal extent)
   a. Lower one-third (Li)
   b. Mid one-third; below tracheal bifurcation (Lm)
   c. Upper one-third; above tracheal bifurcation (Ls)

5. Adjunctive findings
   a. Erosion (E)

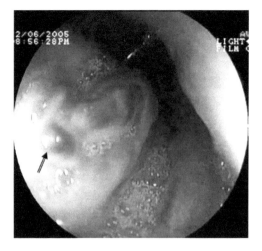

Figure 10.7 "Red wale" mark (arrow) on the varix.

Figure 10.8 Hematocystic spot, i.e., discrete elevated red spot (arrow) on varix.

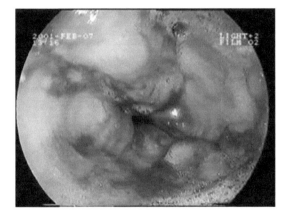

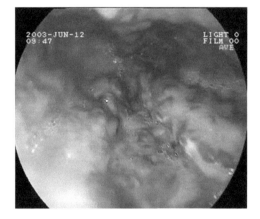

Figure 10.9 Diffuse redness on the varices.

Figure 10.10 Secondary varices, i.e., small tortuous collaterals between main variceal columns.

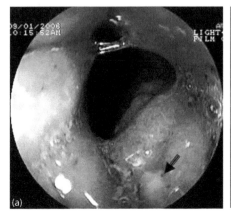

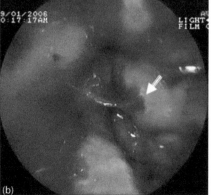

Figure 10.11 **(a, b)** Fibrin plug (arrow) on a varix just below GE junction indicating the site of rupture. (b) During examination, the plug got dislodged and the varix started bleeding actively (arrow).

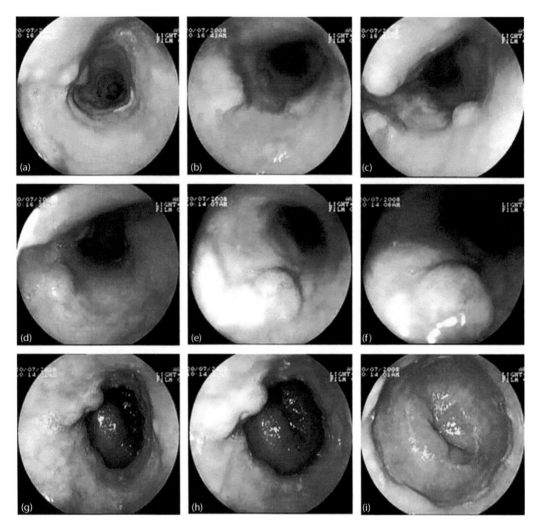

Figure 10.12 Pseudo varix. **(a)** Single column of vein showing focal ectasias. **(b–h)** Further examination revealed multiple ectatic veins in the esophageal wall. **(i)** A normal GE junction ruled out varices due to portal hypertension.

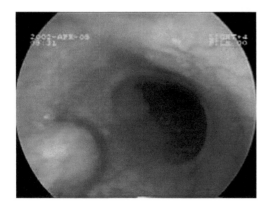

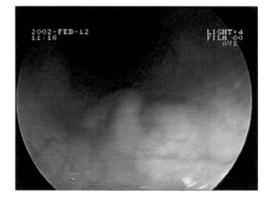

Figure 10.13 Pseudo varix; focal ectasias in a single column of vein in the esophageal wall.

Figure 10.14 Pseudo varix; single column of tortuous vein in mid-esophagus. The GE junction was normal.

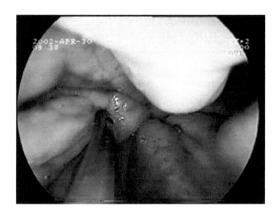

Figure 10.15 Intravariceal sclerotherapy. Sclerosant being injected directly into the varix.

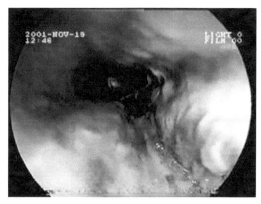

Figure 10.16 Thrombosed varix following sclerotherapy.

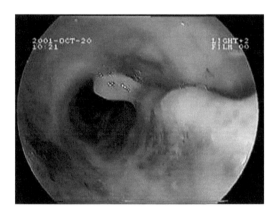

Figure 10.17 Thrombosed varix.

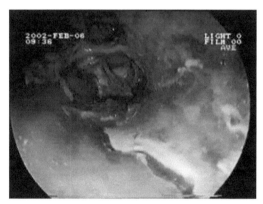

Figure 10.18 Thrombosed varix and ulcerated esophageal mucosa.

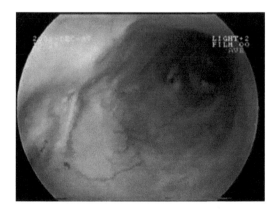

Figure 10.19 Remnants of thrombosed and obliterated varix.

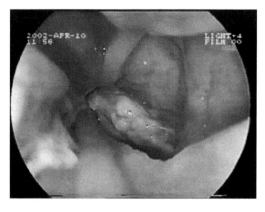

Figure 10.20 Esophageal ulcer following sclerotherapy.

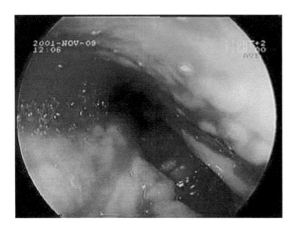

Figure 10.21 Bleeding from post-sclerotherapy esophageal ulcer.

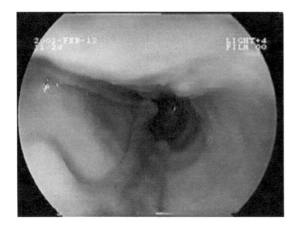

Figure 10.22 Healed post-sclerotherapy ulcer leaving behind irregular mucosa and mucosal tags.

COMPLICATIONS FOLLOWING SCLEROTHERAPY

- General
  - Fever
  - Anaphylaxis
  - Septicemia

- Esophageal
  - Torn varix
  - Retrosternal pain
  - Dysmotility
  - Dysphagia
  - Ulcers
  - Perforation
  - Stricture
  - Squamous cell carcinoma

- Pleuro-pulmonary
  - Atelectasis
  - Pleural effusion
  - Empyema

- Distant
  - Gastric variceal bleeding
  - Bleeding from gastropathy
  - Portal vein periphlebitis
  - Portal vein thrombosis
  - Mesenteric vein thrombosis

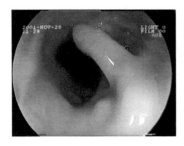

Figure 10.23 Mucosal tag following variceal obliteration.

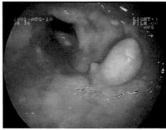

Figure 10.24 Esophageal ulcer and stricture formation following sclerotherapy.

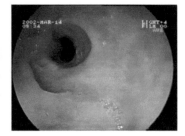

Figure 10.25 Esophageal stricture following sclerotherapy. Varices have been completely eradicated.

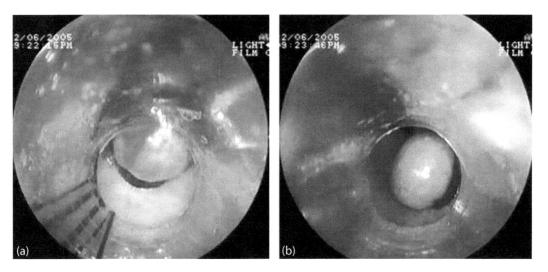

Figure 10.26 **(a, b)** Endoscopic variceal band ligation (EVL). Ligated varix soon after release of the band.

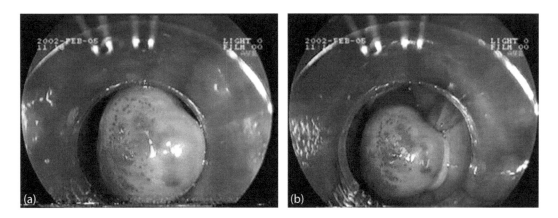

Figure 10.27 **(a, b)** Ligated varix.

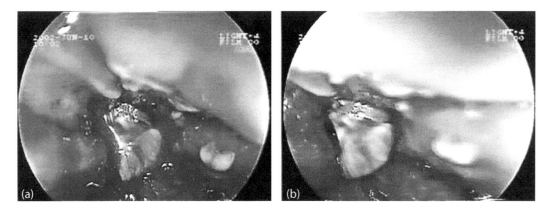

Figure 10.28 **(a, b)** Bleeding from ulcerated varix following EVL.

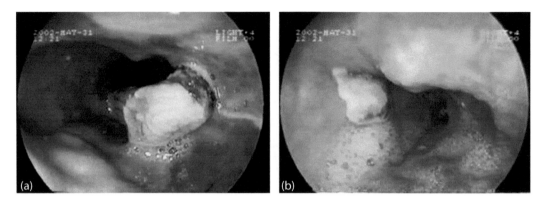

Figure 10.29 Thrombosed and ulcerated varix following EVL. (a) The band is still in place.
(b) The band has fallen off.

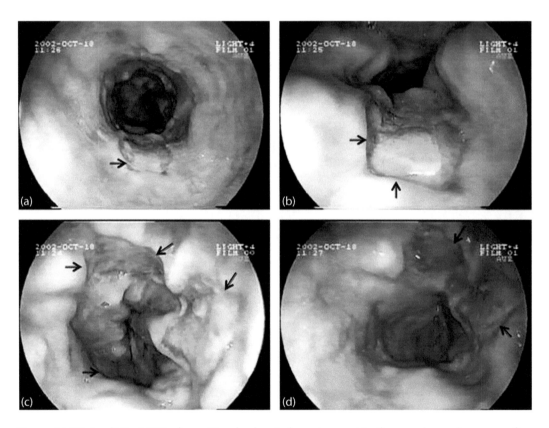

Figure 10.30 (a–d) Post-EVL ulcers. Punched-out ulcers (arrows) in the esophageal mucosa after
sloughing of the thrombosed varices.

Classification of gastric varices

Type	Appearance
1	Varices in the lesser curvature continuous with the esophageal varix.
2	Fundal varices.
3	Both lesser curve and fundal varices.

British Journal Surgery 1990; 77:195.

Type	Appearance
1	Varices appearing as inferior extension of esophageal varices across the squamocolumnar junction.
2	(Nearly always accompanied by esophageal varices) located in the fundus, which appear to converge towards the cardia.
3	Varices located in the fundus or body in the absence of esophageal varices and appear unconnected to the cardia.

British Journal Surgery 1990; 75:195.

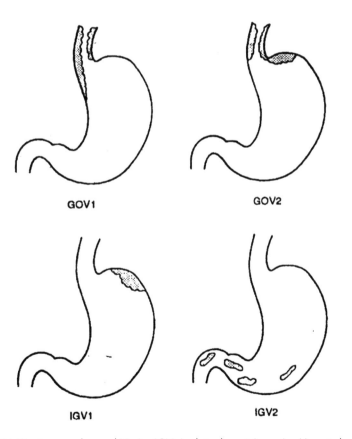

Figure 10.31 GOV: Gastroesophageal Varix; IGV: Isolated gastric varix. *Hepatology* 1992; 16:1343.

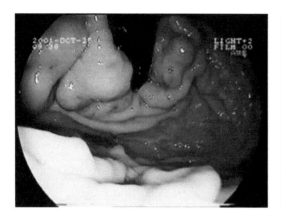

Figure 10.32 Junctional varix. Varices extending from esophagus across the GE junction.

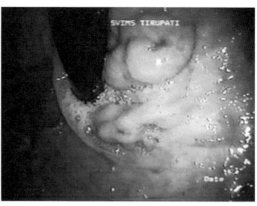

Figure 10.33 Varices just below the GE junction.

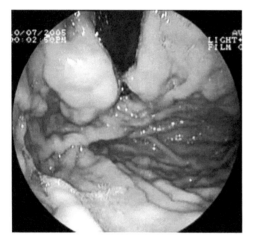

Figure 10.34 Junctional varix.

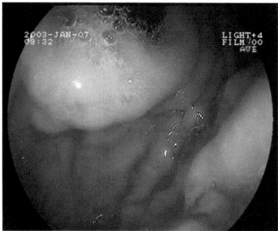

Figure 10.35 Junctional varix.

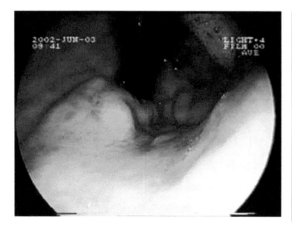

Figure 10.36 Varix extending along the lesser curve.

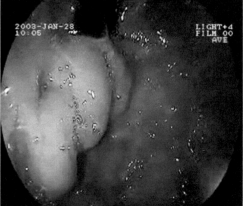

Figure 10.37 Single column of tortuous varix extending along the lesser curve.

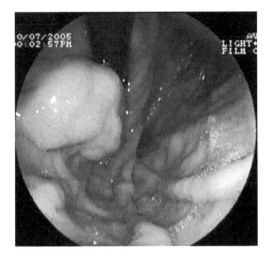

Figure 10.38 Varix below the GE junction.

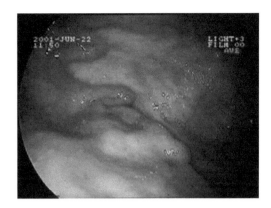

Figure 10.39 Diffuse varix along the lesser curve.

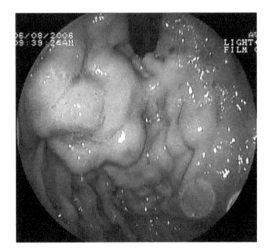

Figure 10.40 Varix below the GE junction.

Figure 10.41 Fundal varix.

Large gastric varices appear like "a bunch of grapes." Small varices should be differentiated from mucosal folds and prominent submucosal veins. Mucosal folds flatten out on distension. Submucosal veins, unlike varices, do not show dilatation or tortuosity.

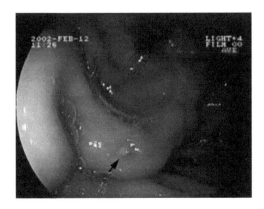

Figure 10.42 "White nipple" sign (arrow) on fundal varix suggesting recent bleeding.

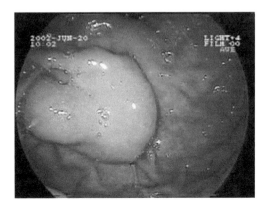

Figure 10.43 Isolated fundal varix.

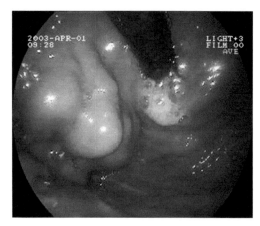

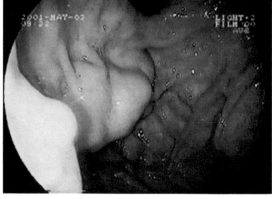

Figure 10.44 Fundal varix.

Figure 10.45 Fundal varix.

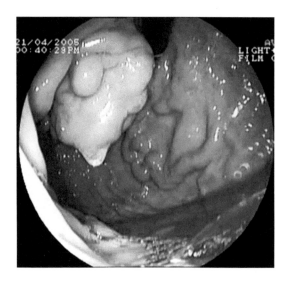

Figure 10.46 Fundal varix appearing like a bunch of grapes.

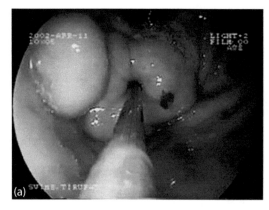

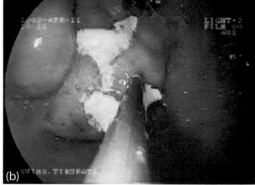

Figure 10.47 (a) Fundal varix being injected with Cyanoacrylate glue. (b) The varix appears rounded due to hardening of the glue inside. Some spilled out glue can be seen on the surface of the varix.

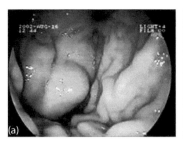
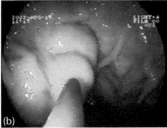
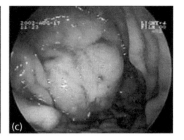

Figure 10.48 **(a)** Large fundal varix. **(b)** cynoacrylate glue injection. **(c)** Solidified varix.

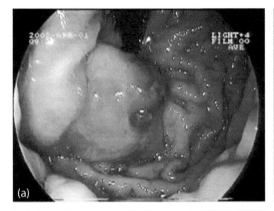
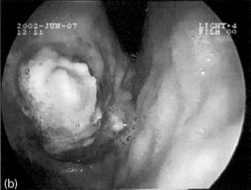

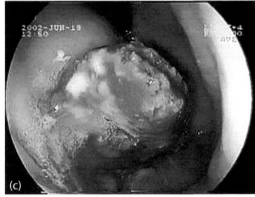

Figure 10.49 **(a)** Ulceration and oozing from the surface of a solidified fundal varix. Cyanoacrylate glue was injected a week earlier. **(b)** About two months later, the ulceration appearing more extensive and the glue extruding out. **(c)** Continued oozing and further extrusion of the glue 12 days later.

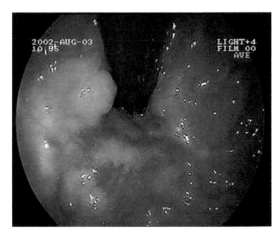

Figure 10.50 Eradicated gastric varix. Scarring and neovascularization in the varix bearing area.

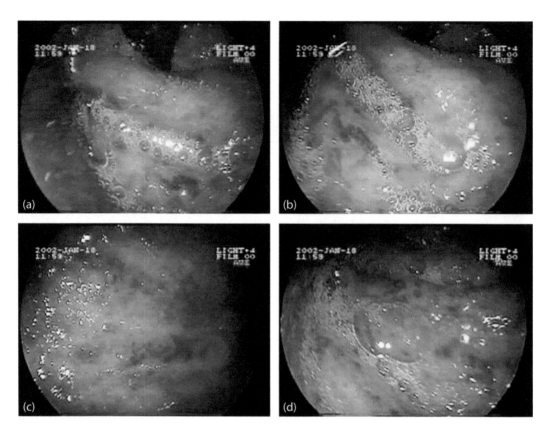

Figure 10.51 (a–d) Appearance of gastric mucosa in portal hypertensive gastropathy.

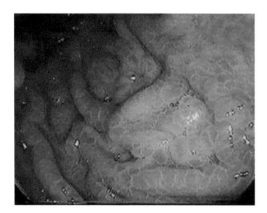

Figure 10.52 Portal hypertensive gastropathy. "Snake-skin" appearance of gastric mucosa.

Portal hypertensive gastropathy (PHG) is most often an incidental finding in patients of portal hypertension. In <2% of patients, it may present with significant upper GI bleeding. The endoscopic appearance of the gastric mucosa in PHG is characterized by a beefy red appearance, petechial hemorrhages, red spots and a mucosal pattern of a white reticular network outlining erythematous central areas (snake-skin appearance). Endoscopic biopsies reveal submucosal edema, dilated submucosal veins, mucosal capillaries and venules. Submucosal arterioles have thickened walls with proliferation of endothelial and adventitial elements. The submucosal venules show morphologic features of arterialization. The overall blood flow to the stomach is increased. There are increased submucosal arteriovenous communications resulting in reduction of effective mucosal blood flow.

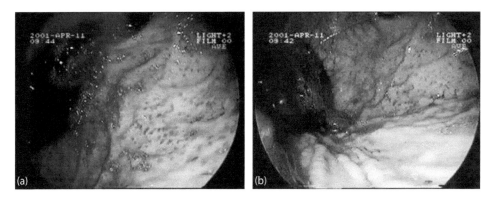

Figure 10.53 (a, b) Mucosal appearance in portal hypertensive gastropathy.

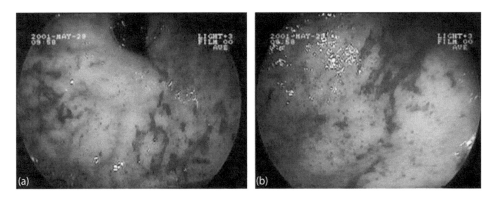

Figure 10.54 (a, b) Bleeding portal hypertensive gastropathy.

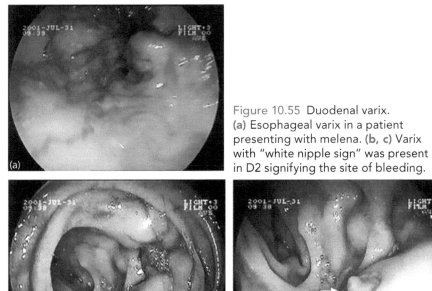

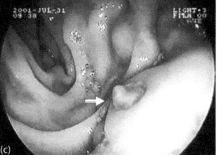

Figure 10.55 Duodenal varix.
(a) Esophageal varix in a patient presenting with melena. (b, c) Varix with "white nipple sign" was present in D2 signifying the site of bleeding.

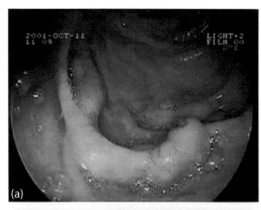

Duodenal varix is found in 0.5%–2.5% of patients with portal hypertension. A higher incidence of 43% has been reported in radiological studies (splenoportogram).

American Journal of Gastroenterology 1993; 88:1942. *Endoscopy* 1996; 28:239. *Radiology* 1968; 8:90.

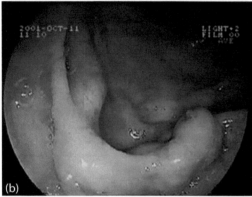

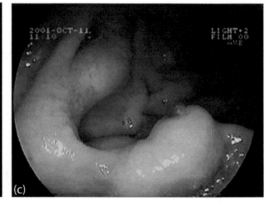

Figure 10.56 (a–c) Ruptured duodenal varix. Solitary varix in D2 showing "white nipple sign."

11

Corrosive injury

In suspected cases of corrosive injury, endoscopy should be performed with utmost care and gentleness following three basic principles: minimal insufflation, avoidance of blind and forceful intubation.

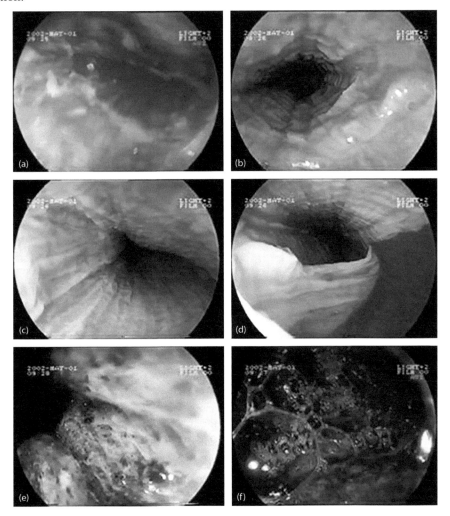

Figure 11.1 Early appearance following acid ingestion. **(a)** Inflamed pharyngeal mucosa. **(b, c)** Thin, whitish membrane covering esophageal mucosa. **(d)** Inflamed mucosa beneath the membrane. **(e, f)** Charred gastric mucosa. *(Continued)*

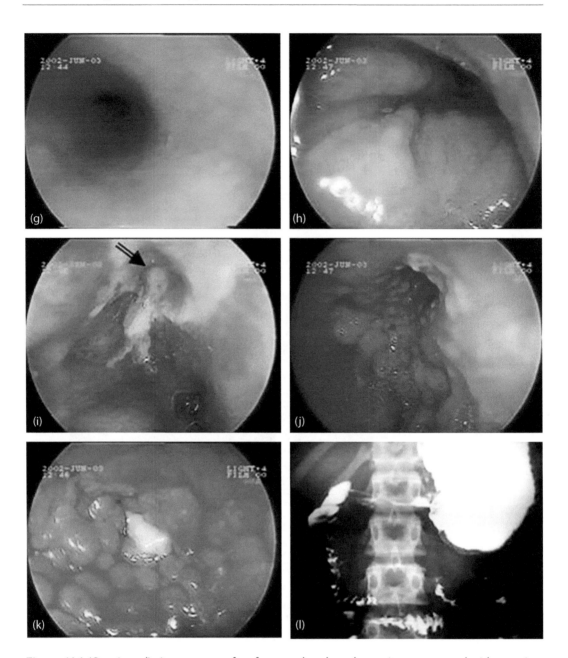

Figure 11.1 (Continued) Appearance after four weeks when the patient presented with gastric outlet obstruction. (g) Healed esophageal mucosa. (h) Inflamed gastric mucosa. (i) Prepyloric antrum showing slough and displaced pylorus (arrow). (j) Removal of slough showing inflamed mucosa. (k) Pyloric channel obscured by slough. (l) Barium study showing contracted antro-pyloric region. The patient was treated with gastrojejunostomy.

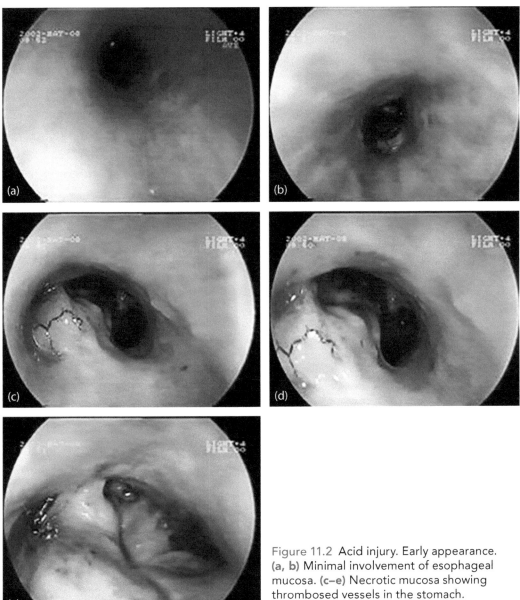

Figure 11.2 Acid injury. Early appearance. (a, b) Minimal involvement of esophageal mucosa. (c–e) Necrotic mucosa showing thrombosed vessels in the stomach.

(Continued)

ENDOSCOPIC GRADING OF CAUSTIC INJURY

Grade 1: Erythema/edema.
Grade 2a: Friability, hemorrhagic blisters, white exudate, superficial ulcers and erythema.
Grade 2b: 2a + deep or circumferential ulcers.
Grade 3a: Small areas of necrosis, brown-black, grayish discoloration, deep ulcers.
Grade 3b: Extensive necrosis.

Gastrointestinal Endoscopy 1991; 37:165

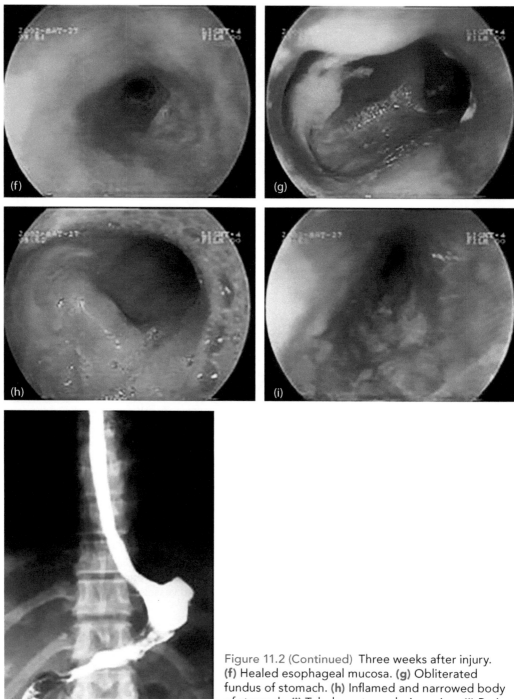

Figure 11.2 (Continued) Three weeks after injury. (f) Healed esophageal mucosa. (g) Obliterated fundus of stomach. (h) Inflamed and narrowed body of stomach. (i) Tubular antro-pyloric region. (j) Barium contrast study of the same patient corroborating the endoscopic findings.

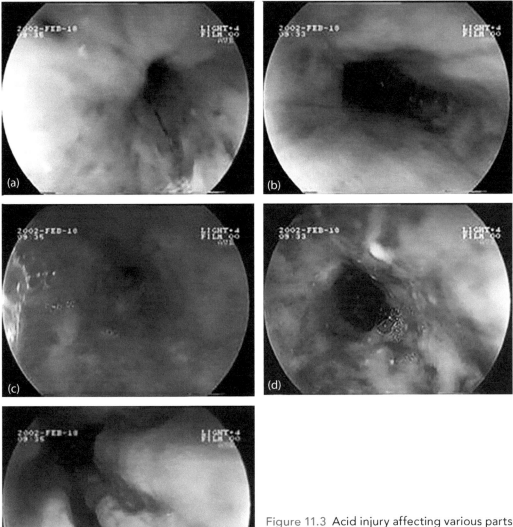

Figure 11.3 Acid injury affecting various parts of the esophagus, appearance in the first 72 h. **(a)** Esophagus just distal to cricopharyngeal opening. **(b–e)** Esophageal mucosa from proximal to distal segment. *(Continued)*

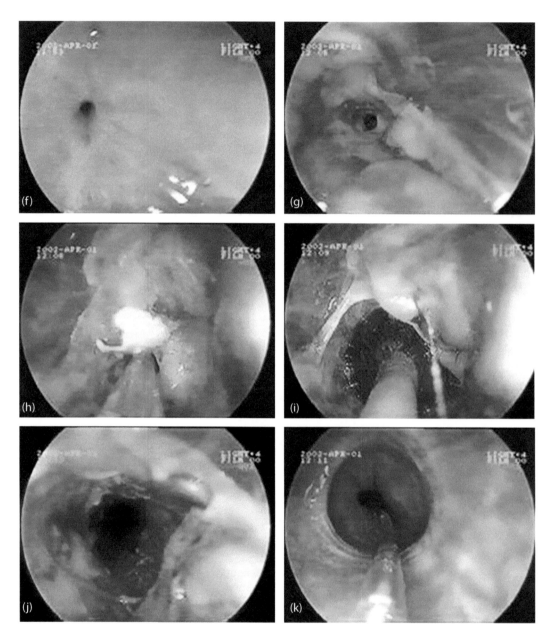

Figure 11.3 (Continued) Six weeks after the injury. (f) Tight stricture in the mid-esophagus. (g–j) Stricture opened up by balloon dilatation. (k) Distal end, relatively healthy.

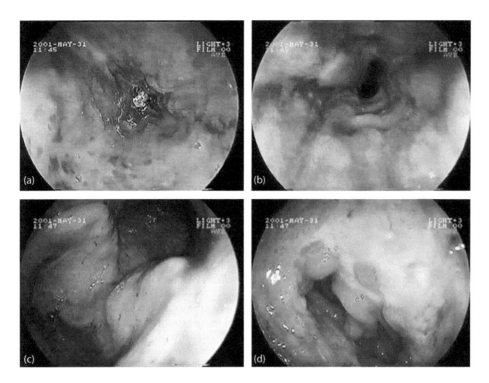

Figure 11.4 Acid injury. (a) Proximal esophageal mucosa. (b) Distal esophageal mucosa. (c) Thick eschar covering gastric body. (d) Inflamed antral mucosa.

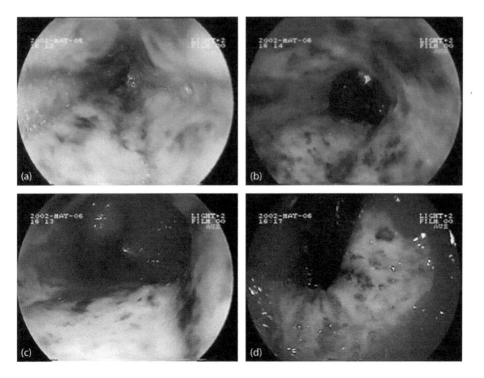

Figure 11.5 (a, b) Acid injury to esophageal mucosa. (c) Note the hiatal hernia and the relatively healthy gastric mucosa in the hernial sac. (d) Same as seen on retroflexion.

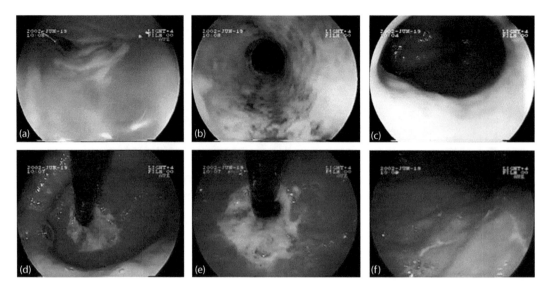

Figure 11.6 Chemical burn in a patient who consumed spurious alcohol 24 h earlier. **(a)** Superficial burn involving pharynx and **(b)** esophagus. **(c)** Hiatal hernia in the same patient. **(d)** Retroflex view showing the hiatal sac and the junction of the affected esophageal mucosa and normal gastric mucosa. **(e)** Close-up view of the same. **(f)** Multiple superficial ulcers in the gastric body.

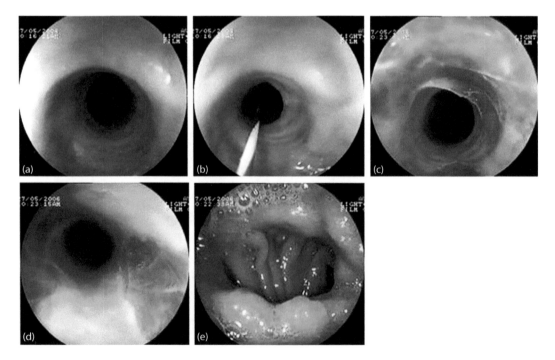

Figure 11.7 **(a)** Corrosive stricture in the mid-esophagus. **(b)** Guidewire across the stricture. **(c, d)** Stricture bearing segment after dilatation. **(e)** Gastrojejunostomy in the same patient performed earlier for antral stricture.

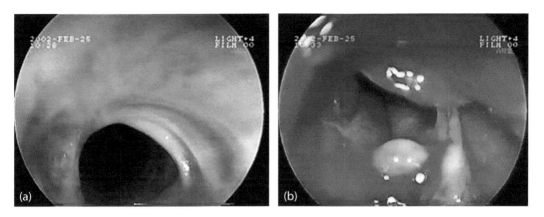

Figure 11.8 **(a)** Corrosive stricture involving mid-esophagus. **(b)** Same after balloon dilatation.

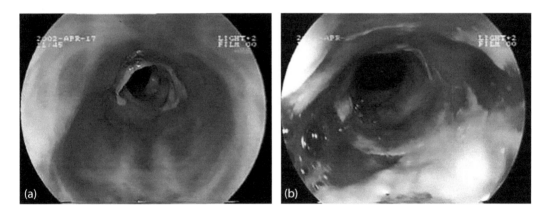

Figure 11.9 Corrosive stricture **(a)** before and **(b)** after dilatation.

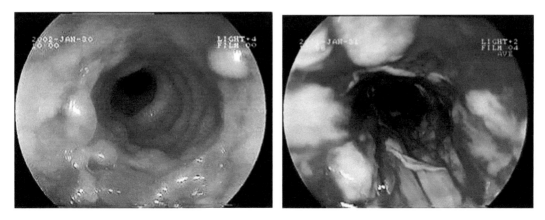

Figure 11.10 Corrosive stricture.

Figure 11.11 Corrosive stricture after dilatation.

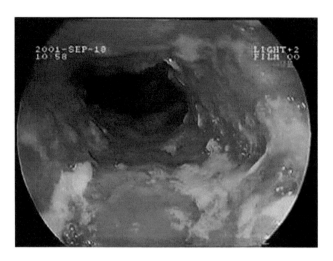

Figure 11.12 Corrosive stricture after dilatation.

12

Uncommon inflammatory lesions and tropical diseases of the UGI tract

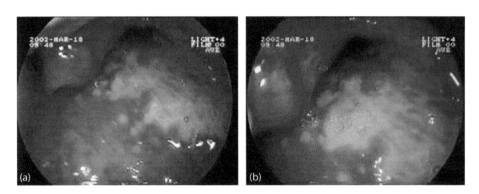

Figure 12.1 **(a, b)** Pharyngeal ulcers in an immunocompromised patient.

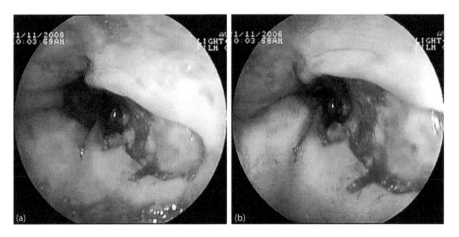

Figure 12.2 **(a, b)** Human immunodeficiency virus (HIV)–associated idiopathic ulcer in the mid-esophagus.

Esophageal involvement in HIV-infected patients can be

- Fungal: *Candida*
- Viral: Cytomegalovirus (CMV), herpes simplex virus (HSV)
- Idiopathic

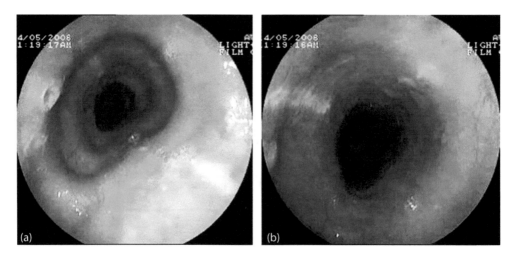

Figure 12.3 **(a, b)** Herpes simplex virus (HSV) ulcers in the mid-esophagus showing minimal involvement.

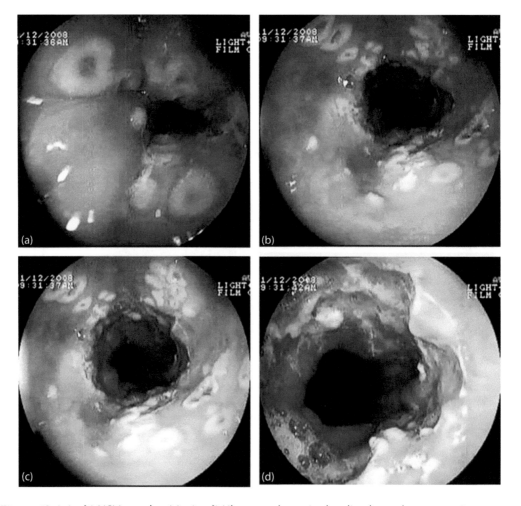

Figure 12.4 **(a, b)** HSV esophagitis. **(c, d)** Ulcers coalesce in the distal esophagus causing mucosal necrosis

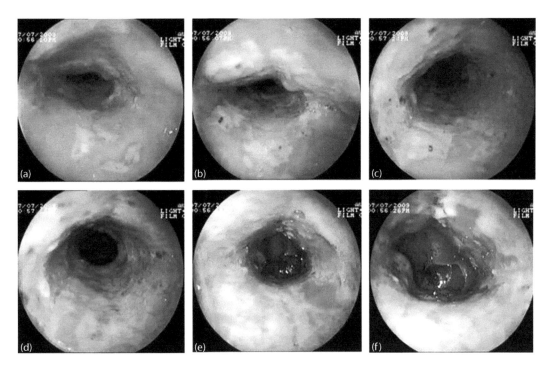

Figure 12.5 HSV esophagitis. **(a)** Discrete ulcers in the proximal esophagus. **(b–f)** Ulcers coalesce distally to cause circumferential involvement.

HSV esophagitis commonly presents with acute onset dysphagia, odynophagia and chest pain. On endoscopy, the ulcers appear sharply demarcated, having raised margins. Typically known as "volcano ulcers," they may coalesce to cause confluent ulcers.

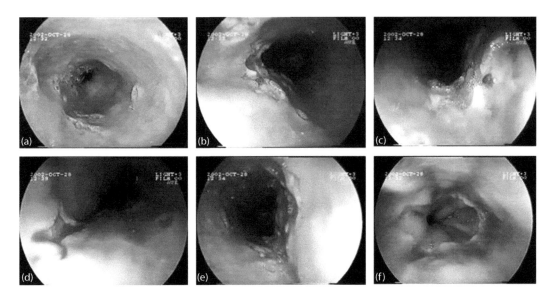

Figure 12.6 **(a–e)** CMV esophageal ulcers. These ulcers are deep, having irregular borders and finger-like projections. **(f)** The distal esophagus appears normal.

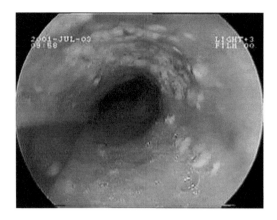

Figure 12.7 *Candida* esophagitis.

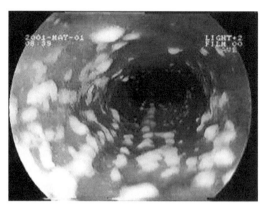

Figure 12.8 *Candida* esophagitis.

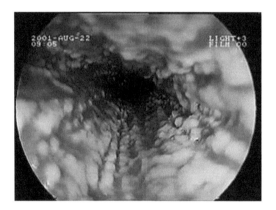

Figure 12.9 *Candida* esophagitis.

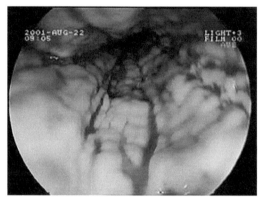

Figure 12.10 *Candida* esophagitis.

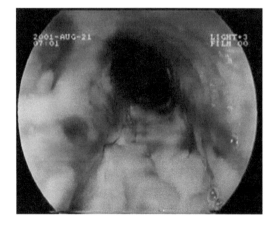

Figure 12.11 *Candida* esophagitis.

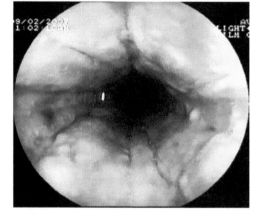

Figure 12.12 *Candida* esophagitis.

PREDISPOSING FACTORS FOR *CANDIDA* ESOPHAGITIS

Immunosuppression, diabetes mellitus, corticosteroid therapy, prolonged antibiotics, esophageal obstruction and malignancy.

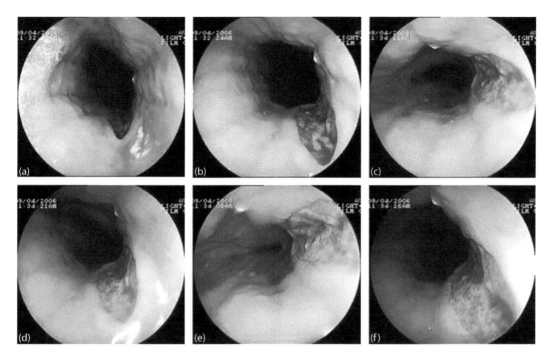

Figure 12.13 (a–f) Esophageal ulcer in Behcet's disease.

Gastrointestinal involvement occurs in 3%–16% of patients with Behcet's disease. The esophagus and the ileocecal region are the two most common sites of involvement.

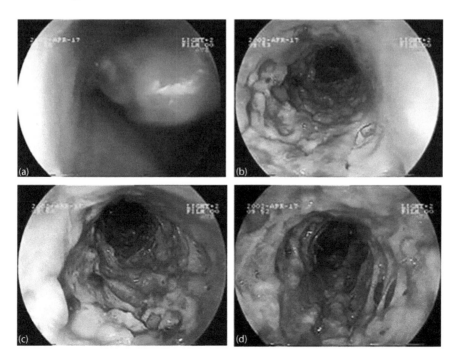

Figure 12.14 Granulomatous sarcoma of the esophagus. Myeloid cell infiltration of the esophageal mucosa in a patient with acute myeloid leukemia. (a) Ulcer in the epiglottis. (b–e) Nodular and ulcerated mucosa with slough involving the entire esophagus. (f) No involvement beyond the Z line. (Continued)

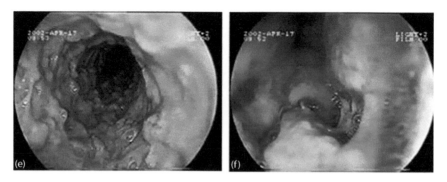

Figure 12.14 (Continued) Granulomatous sarcoma of the esophagus. Myeloid cell infiltration of the esophageal mucosa in a patient with acute myeloid leukemia. **(a)** Ulcer in the epiglottis. **(b–e)** Nodular and ulcerated mucosa with slough involving the entire esophagus. **(f)** No involvement beyond the Z line.

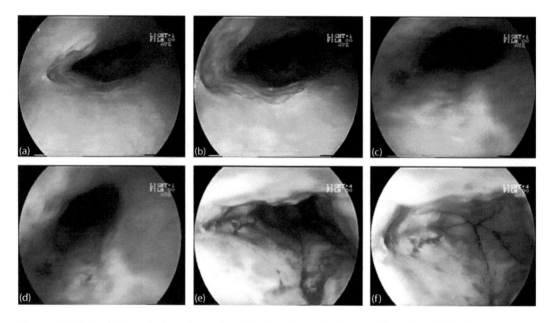

Figure 12.15 **(a–f)** Drug-induced esophagitis. Esophageal ulcers and erosions following doxycycline ingestion the previous day.

DRUGS COMMONLY CAUSING ESOPHAGEAL INJURY

NSAIDs	Vitamin C	Tetracyclines	Doxycycline
Potassium Chloride	Ferrous Sulfate	Quinine Sulfate	Quinidine
Zidovudine			

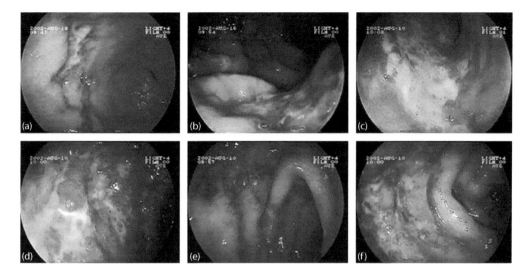

Figure 12.16 Acute infectious gastroduodenitis. **(a, b)** Multiple ulcers in the gastric antrum **(c, d)** in D1 and **(e, f)** in the descending duodenum. The patient presented with acute abdominal pain, vomiting and fever. Mucosal biopsy was nonspecific. Such ulcers were possibly infective in origin. The symptoms resolved on conservative treatment spanning over two weeks.

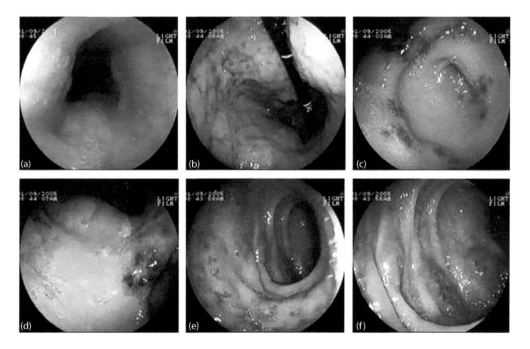

Figure 12.17 Acute infectious gastroduodenitis. **(a)** Normal-appearing esophagus and **(b)** fundus. **(c, d)** Multiple ulcers in the antrum and around the pylorus. **(e)** Ulcers in D1 and **(f)** D2. Patient, a 13-year-old boy presented with acute abdominal pain, fever, loose motion and melena. He was empirically treated with oral omeprazole and ciprofloxacin. *(Continued)*

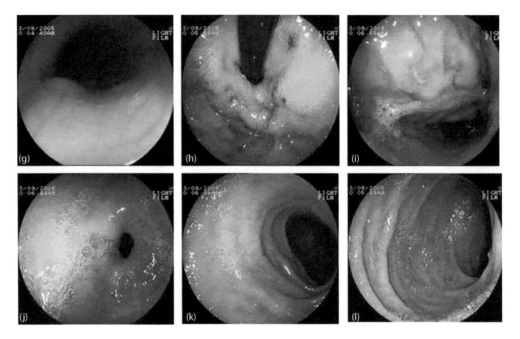

Figure 12.17 (Continued) Endoscopy 12 days later for persistent symptoms showed **(a)** normal esophagus, **(h, i)** mucosal edema and ulceration involving the fundus and body. Ulcers in **(j)** antrum, **(k)** D1 and **(l)** D2 showing signs of healing. *(Continued)*

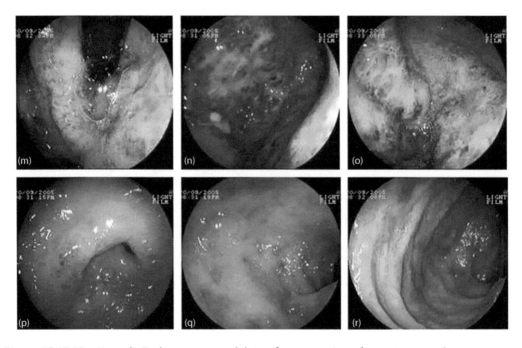

Figure 12.17 (Continued) Endoscopy a week later, for worsening of symptoms and hematemesis, showed diffuse mucosal ulcerations involving **(m)** fundus, **(n, o)** body, **(p)** antrum, **(q)** D1 and **(r)** D2. Mucosal biopsy from the lesions showed nonspecific inflammation. Serum gastrin level was normal. The patient was treated with an anti–*H. pylori* regimen (pantoprazole, clarithromycin and metronidazole). *(Continued)*

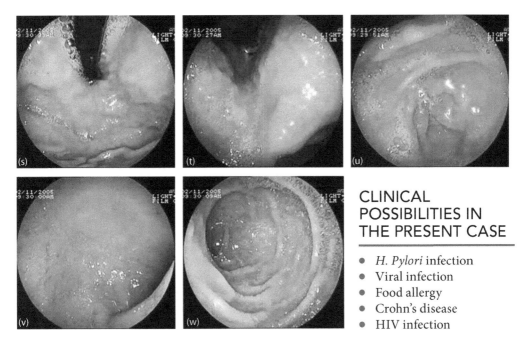

CLINICAL POSSIBILITIES IN THE PRESENT CASE

- *H. Pylori* infection
- Viral infection
- Food allergy
- Crohn's disease
- HIV infection

Figure 12.17 (Continued) Endoscopy two months later showed slight mucosal irregularity suggestive of healed ulcers in (s) fundus, (t) body and (u) antrum. Complete mucosal healing was observed in (v) D1 and (w) D2.

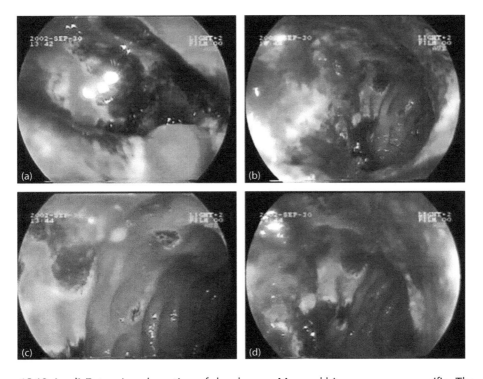

Figure 12.18 (a–d) Extensive ulceration of duodenum. Mucosal biopsy was nonspecific. The patient presented with acute abdominal pain, fever and bloody diarrhea. The symptoms resolved nearly three weeks after conservative management with antibiotics and proton pump inhibitors. The disease possibly represented idiopathic segmental enteritis.

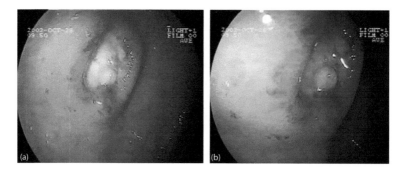

Figure 12.19 **(a, b)** Duodenal tuberculosis. Ulcer on the anterior wall at the junction of D1 and D2. The patient presented with low-grade fever and weight loss. Biopsy of the ulcer margin showed caseating granuloma.

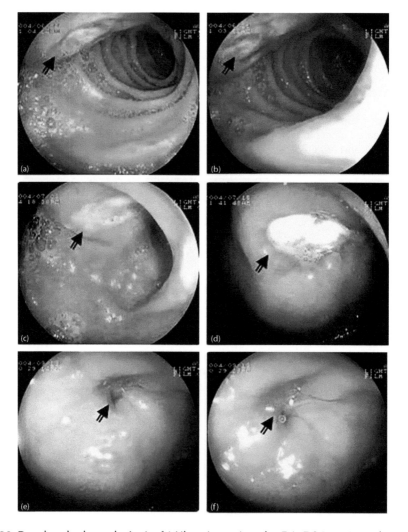

Figure 12.20 Duodenal tuberculosis. **(a, b)** Ulcer (arrow) at the D1–D2 junction. The patient was started on proton pump inhibitors. **(c, d)** Repeat endoscopy about three weeks later showed no signs of healing; instead the ulcer seemed to have worsened. Ulcer biopsy at this stage suggested tuberculosis. **(e, f)** Endoscopy about one month after starting antituberculosis treatment. The ulcer (arrow) showed marked reduction in size. The patient received the full course of antituberculosis treatment.

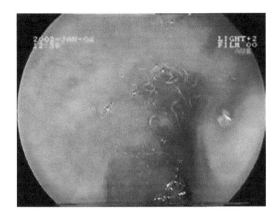

Figure 12.21 Pinworms in D1.

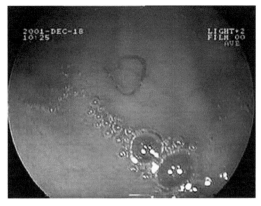

Figure 12.22 Hookworm in D1.

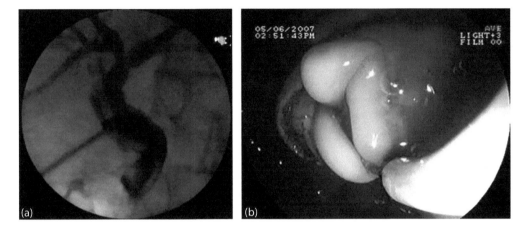

Figure 12.23 Biliary ascariasis. (a) T-tube cholangiogram showing an *Ascaris lumbricoides* (roundworm) in the bile duct. (b) The worm was delivered out by a snare after endoscopic sphincterotomy.

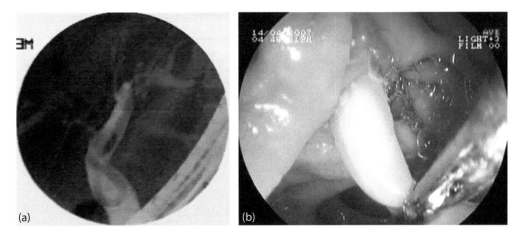

Figure 12.24 Endoscopic retrograde cholangiogram showing a roundworm in the proximal biliary tree. (b) The worm was extracted after grasping it with endoscopic "rat tooth" forceps.

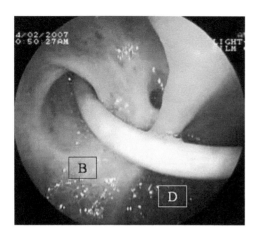

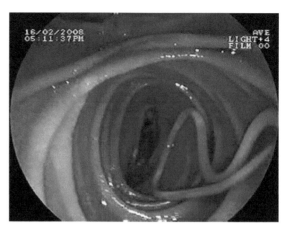

Figure 12.25 Roundworm across a choledochoduodenostomy stoma. Note the bile duct lumen (B) and the duodenum (D).

Figure 12.26 Roundworm in D3.

13

Mallory–Weiss syndrome

Mallory–Weiss syndrome accounts for 5%–10% of all cases of upper gastrointestinal bleeding. The typical presentation is frank hematemesis or blood streaking of vomitus that follows normal bouts of vomiting occurring in the setting of alcoholism, food poisoning or hyperemesis gravidarum. On endoscopy, it is characterized by one or more linear mucosal tear involving the GE junction. The tear may extend for variable distance onto the GE junction. Bleeding from such a lesion is usually mild and self-limiting and responds to conservative management. Endoscopic intervention, in the form of local adrenaline saline injection, thermal coagulation, hemoclip application or banding may be required in the rare event of continued bleeding.

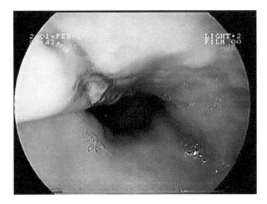

Figure 13.1 Linear tear at the 10-o'clock position.

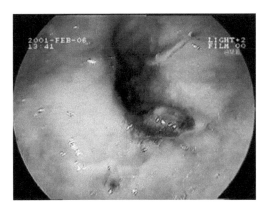

Figure 13.2 Linear tears at the two- and five-o'clock positions.

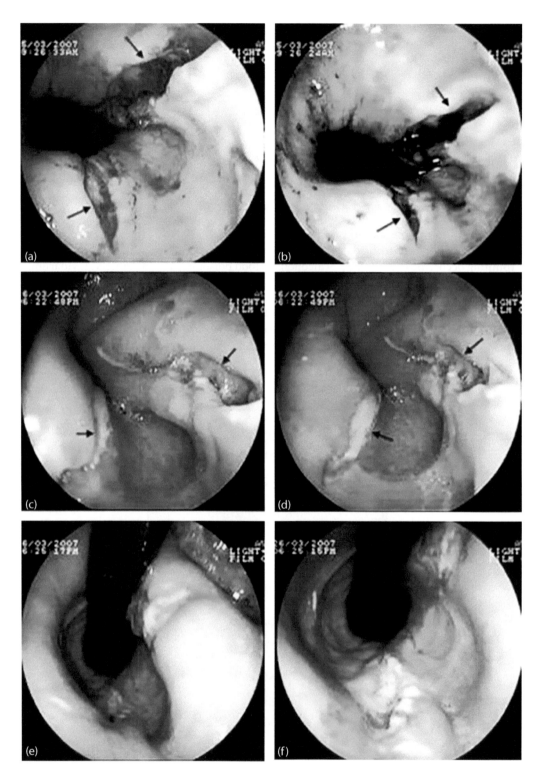

Figure 13.3 (a, b) Linear lacerations (arrows) across the GE junction. The patient presented with massive hematemesis following an alcoholic binge. (c, d) Repeat endoscopy 24 h later; the altered blood in the lesion has been replaced by whitish slough. Note the sliding hiatal hernia. (e, f) Lacerations extending on to gastric mucosa beyond the hiatal sac as seen on retroflexion.

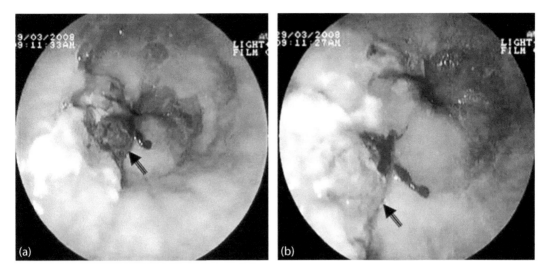

Figure 13.4 **(a, b)** Lacerated esophageal mucosa and submucosal hematoma (arrow) at the Z line.

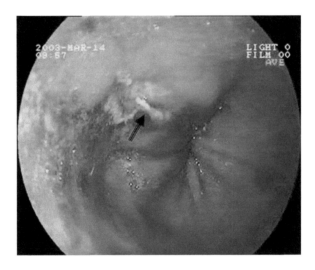

Figure 13.5 A linear tear at the GE junction.

Dieulafoy's lesion

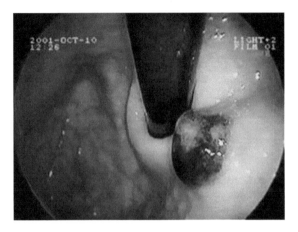

Figure 14.1 Dieulafoy's lesion just below GE junction seen on retroflexion.

Dieulafoy's lesion (exulceratio simplex, caliber-persistent artery) is characterized by the presence of a thick-caliber submucosal arteriole that can cause torrential bleeding. This lesion most commonly occurs in the proximal 6 cm of the stomach. Less commonly, it may occur in the duodenum and the rest of the GI tract. Endoscopic appearance of duodenal Dieulafoy's lesion ranges from a pinpoint dot, clot or tortuous vessel to blood oozing or spurting from normal mucosa. Management includes injection sclerotherapy, monopolar or bipolar heater probe application, laser photocoagulation, band ligation, application of hemoclip or surgical excision.

Digestive Diseases and Sciences 1988; 33:801

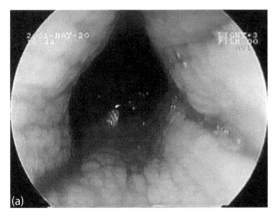
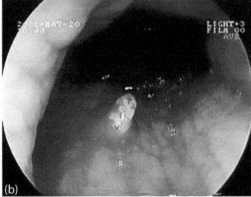

Figure 14.2 **(a, b)** Actively bleeding Dieulafoy's lesion in the body of the stomach. The bleeding point appeared exaggerated because of the adherent fibrin plug and clot.

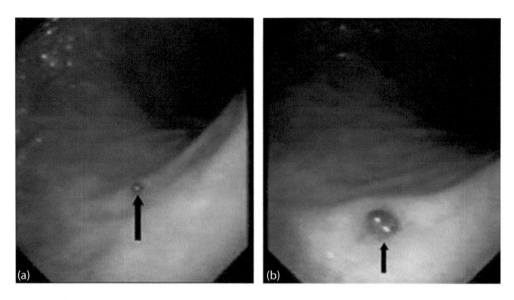

Figure 14.3 (a, b) Dieulafoy's lesion in the proximal stomach appearing as a tiny protuberance. The patient had massive hematemesis 48 h earlier.

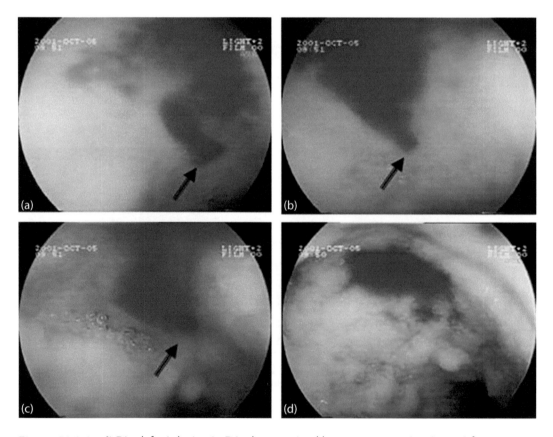

Figure 14.4 (a–d) Dieulafoy's lesion in D1, characterized by punctate oozing (arrow) from an otherwise normal mucosa. Patient, a young woman, presented with recurrent melena.

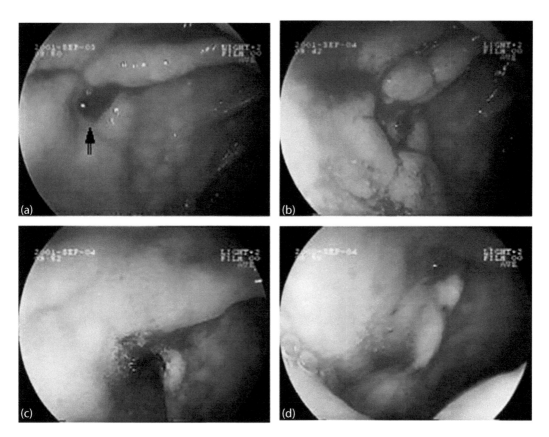

Figure 14.5 (a) Dieulafoy's lesion, quiescent at the time of examination, is covered with a small clot and blood pool (arrow). Note the surrounding normal mucosa that differentiates it from chronic duodenal ulcer. (b) Repeat examination the following day showed an actively bleeding lesion. (c, d) Bleeding was controlled with adrenaline injection.

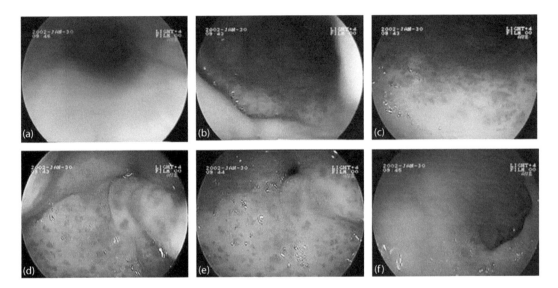

Gastric antral vascular ectasia (GAVE)

Figure 15.1 Gastric antral vascular ectasia (GAVE). **(a)** Normal esophagus. **(b, c)** Punctate telangiectasias confined to the antrum **(d, e)** Close-up view of the same. **(f)** Normal duodenum.

Gastric antral vascular ectasia (GAVE) accounts for nearly 4% of non-variceal UGI bleeding. The entity commonly occurs in association with chronic liver disease, chronic renal failure, autoimmune connective tissue disorder, bone marrow transplantation, ischemic or valvular heart disease, hypertension, familial Mediterranean anemia and acute myeloid anemia. The pathogenesis of the entity is not clearly understood. The presentation ranges from occult to frank GI bleeding. Two types of lesions have been identified on endoscopy: punctuate or striped. Because of similarity in appearance, the striped variety is also known as "watermelon" stomach. Though the antral region shows predominant involvement, occasionally it may extend to the gastric fundus as well. In chronic liver disease, it must be differentiated from portal hypertensive gastropathy as the treatment modalities for both are quite different. Unlike PHG, reduction in portal pressure has no effect on GAVE. Argon plasma coagulation, laser photocoagulation and heater probe application are the accepted modalities of treatment. Rarely, antrectomy may be required for uncontrolled hemorrhage.

Digestion 2008; 77: 131

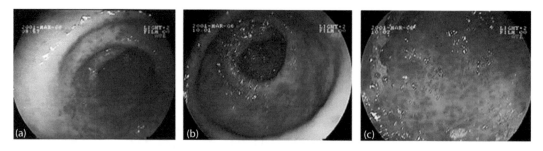

Figure 15.2 **(a, b)** Punctate variety of GAVE. **(c)** Close-up view of the same.

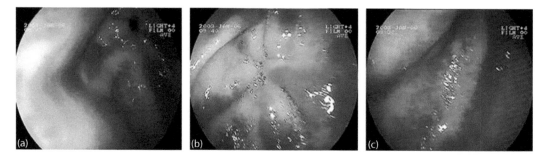

Figure 15.3 Gastric antral vascular ectasia (watermelon stomach). **(a, b)** Linear disposition of vascular ectasias, confined to the antrum, resemble the stripes of a watermelon. **(c)** Close-up view of the same.

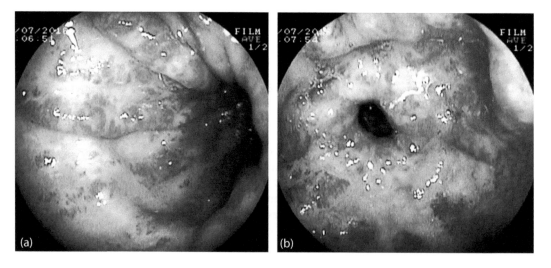

Figure 15.4 Gastric antral vascular ectasia. **(a, b)** Linear telangiectasias confined to the antrum. The patient, a 45-year-old woman, presented with recurrent episodes of melena.

16

Foreign body

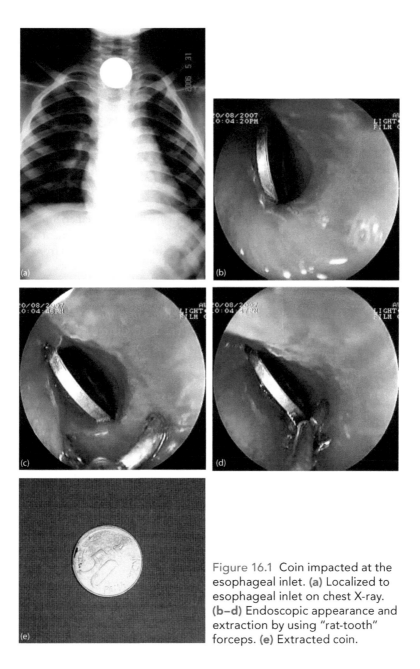

Figure 16.1 Coin impacted at the esophageal inlet. **(a)** Localized to esophageal inlet on chest X-ray. **(b–d)** Endoscopic appearance and extraction by using "rat-tooth" forceps. **(e)** Extracted coin.

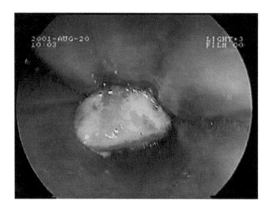

Figure 16.2 Betel nut, swallowed accidentally, lodged at the distal esophagus in a child.

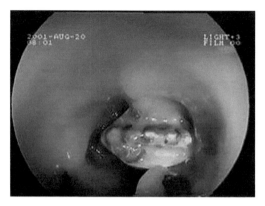

Figure 16.3 A metal ring impacted at the esophageal inlet.

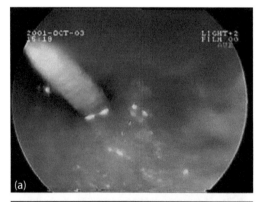

(a)

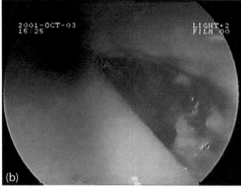

(b)

Figure 16.4 (a) A coin impacted at the esophageal inlet (cricopharyngeal sphincter). (b) Deep mucosal ulcer at the site of impaction, as seen after the coin was extracted.

Esophageal inlet is the commonest site of foreign body (FB) impaction. Dysphagia, odynophagia, chest pain and excessive salivation are the usual symptoms. Contrary to the common practice, FB extraction should always be performed under general anesthesia. It is our practice to use intravenous propofol anesthesia in adults and intubation anesthesia in the pediatric age group. A quiet patient, relaxed cricopharyngeus, secure airway and proper instrument are paramount in successful removal of a FB from the UGI tract.

MANAGEMENT GUIDELINES

Food bolus in esophagus: Remove urgently if the patient is in distress. Remove electively if the patient is comfortable, but do not delay beyond 24 h.

FB in esophagus: Endoscopy and removal as early as possible.

Smooth, rounded FB in stomach: Normal passage is expected in four to six days, but may take up to four weeks. Endoscopic removal is recommended for objects more than 2.5 cm in diameter or longer than 6–10 cm or remaining in the stomach for more than four weeks.

Sharp/pointed objects in stomach: Remove urgently. If it has gone beyond the duodenum, expectant but watchful management is advocated for any signs of obstruction, perforation or bleeding. Remove if it does not pass out in 72 h.

Button battery: Follow if it has gone beyond esophagus. Active removal is indicated for battery more than 2 cm in diameter, age <5 y or if it remains in stomach for more than 48 h.

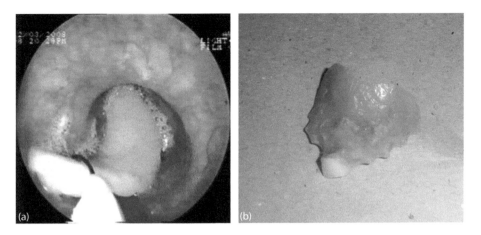

Figure 16.5 (a) Denture impacted at cricopharyngeal sphincter held by a snare. (b) After its extraction.

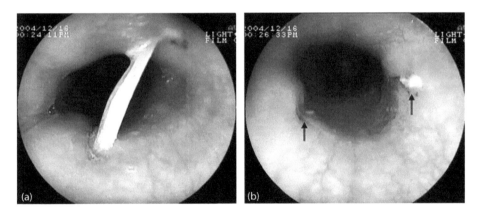

Figure 16.6 (a) A fish bone across the mid-esophagus (b) mucosal injury at the sites of impaction (arrows) seen after its endoscopic removal.

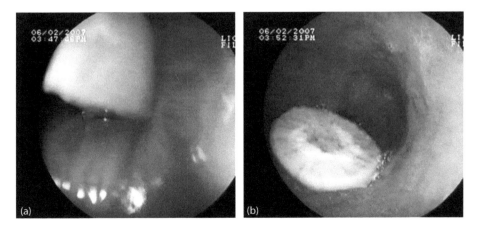

Figure 16.7 (a) A piece of salad (vegetable slice) impacted at the esophageal inlet and (b) dislodged and pushed to the distal esophagus by endoscopic manipulation.

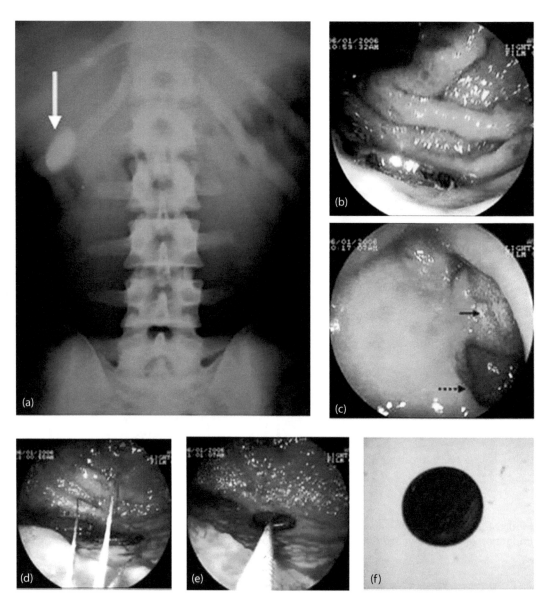

Figure 16.8 A coin swallowed two years back. (a) Localized to the upper abdomen (arrow) on X-ray. (b) On endoscopy, the coin was found to be in the stomach. Such a rounded object should have, in normal circumstances, passed out in a 24–48 h period. The persistence of the object in the stomach was due to chronic duodenal ulcer leading to narrowed outlet. (c) Note the deformed duodenal bulb, an active ulcer (arrow) and pseudodiverticulum (broken arrow). (d, e) The coin was extracted with the help of a Dormia basket. (f) The extracted coin appeared completely blackened due to the prolonged contact with the gastric secretions.

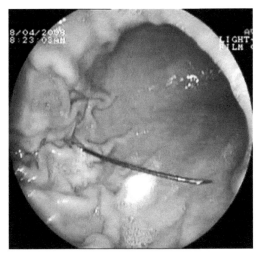

Figure 16.9 A needle at the junction of the body and the antrum.

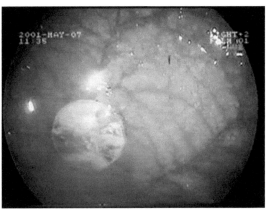

Figure 16.10 A coin in the fundus of the stomach.

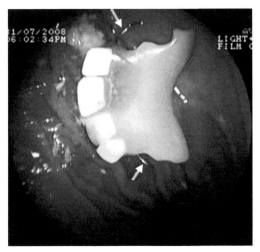

Figure 16.11 Accidentally swallowed denture in the stomach. Its quadrangular shape and the two spikes (arrows) make its endoscopic extraction extremely difficult and risky. Gastrotomy and removal is our preferred approach for such an object.

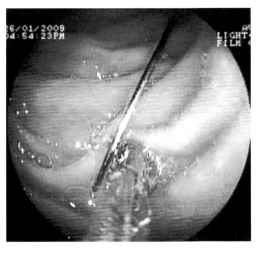

Figure 16.12 A needle in the second part of duodenum. It was held at its proximal end and delivered out along with the endoscope. Holding the needle in such manner is essential to avoid mucosal trauma.

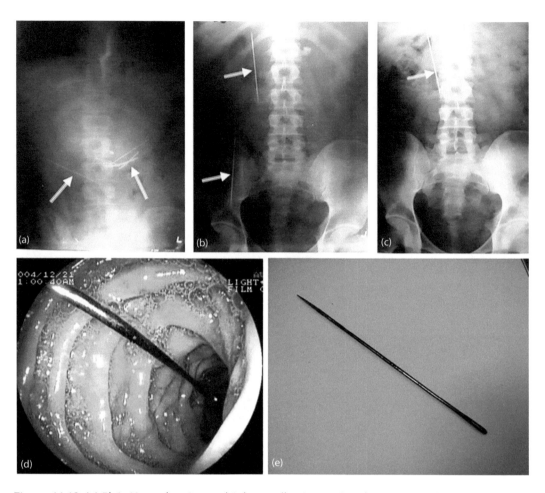

Figure 16.13 **(a)** Plain X-ray showing multiple needles (arrows) in the GI tract. The patient, an adult with a mental illness, was habitually swallowing sewing needles. **(b)** Two needles (arrows), the upper one possibly in the descending duodenum. The patient was fortunate to pass out the needles without any complications. **(c)** Needle persisting in the duodenum. **(d)** Endoscopic view of the same. **(e)** The needle after its extraction.

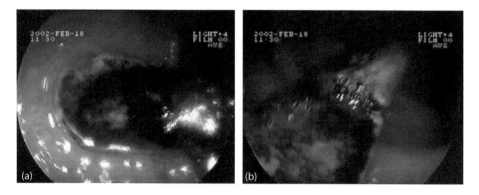

Figure 16.14 **(a, b)** A bile-stained tongue cleaner in descending duodenum. This was accidentally swallowed by the patient about two months back. Endoscopy was done for dyspeptic symptoms.

17

Tracheoesophageal fistula

Tracheoesophageal fistula (TEF) can be congenital or acquired.

ETIOLOGY OF ACQUIRED FISTULA

- Benign
  - Pressure necrosis by the cuff of endotracheal/tracheostomy tube
  - Penetrating injury
  - Erosion by impacted foreign body
  - Erosion by caseating mediastinal lymph node
- Malignant
  - Locally advanced carcinoma
  - Mediastinal lymphoma after irradiation

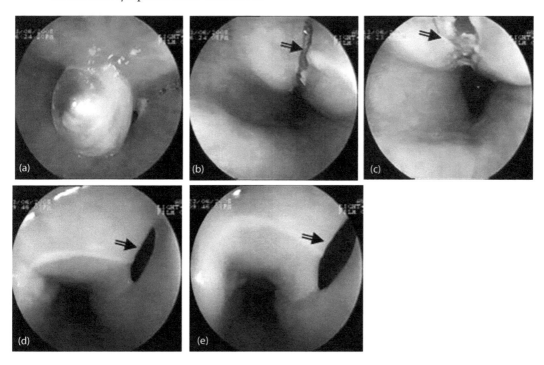

Figure 17.1 Benign TEF arising from pressure necrosis by the inflated tracheostomy cuff.
(a) Bubbling of tracheal secretion through the fistula. (b, c) A rent (arrow) was seen in the cervical esophagus at 12-o'clock position. The transparent tracheostomy cuff is visible through the rent.
(d, e) The same rent (arrow) after removal of the tracheostomy tube.

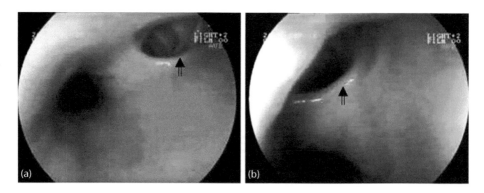

Figure 17.2 **(a, b)** Benign TEF consequent upon pressure necrosis by the inflated cuff of tracheostomy tube. The tracheal opening (arrow) was visible upon entering the cervical esophagus. Note the concentric tracheal rings.

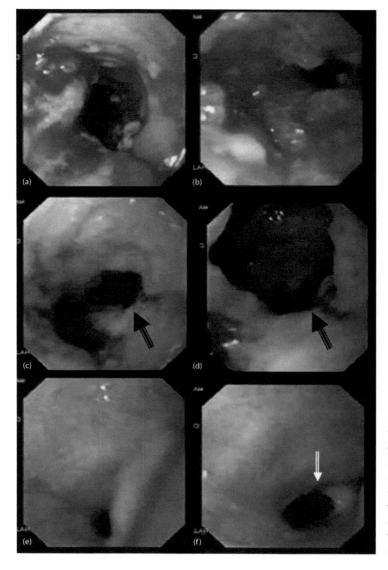

Figure 17.3 Malignant TEF. **(a, b)** Friable tumor involving cervical esophagus. **(c, d)** Tracheal opening (arrow) was visible while maneuvering the endoscope in the esophagus. **(e, f)** Closer view revealed the tracheal rings (white arrow).

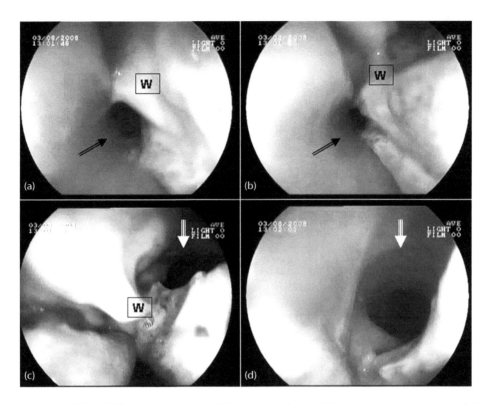

Figure 17.4 **(a–d)** TEF following necrosis of the intervening wall between the trachea and the esophagus. The patient, a young man, had received radiotherapy for mediastinal lymphoma. Note the esophageal lumen (black arrow), the necrotic wall (W) and the trachea (white arrow).

18

Miscellaneous

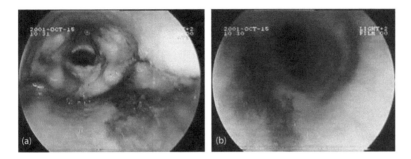

Figure 18.1 **(a)** Pigmentation involving the pharynx, the larynx and **(b)** the esophagus. Incidental finding in an otherwise normal individual.

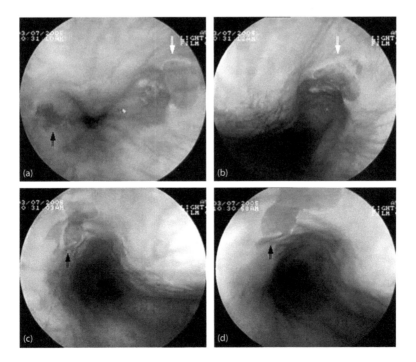

Figure 18.2 "Inlet Patch." **(a)** Islands of heterotropic gastric mucosa (arrows) in the proximal esophagus. **(b)** Patch on the right side. **(c, d)** Close-up view of the patch on the left side. This is usually an incidental finding and has no clinical significance.

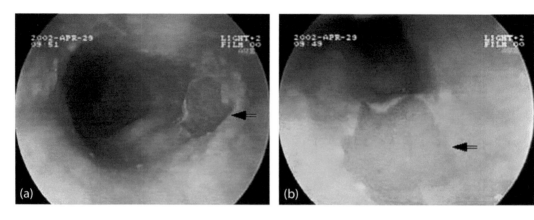

Figure 18.3 **(a, b)** "Inlet patch" (arrow) in the proximal esophagus.

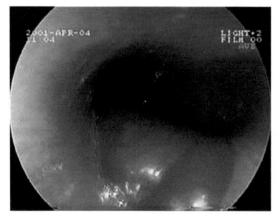

Figure 18.4 Spontaneous esophageal hematoma.

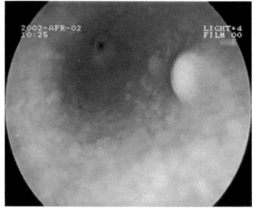

Figure 18.5 Glycogen acanthoma in the esophageal body.

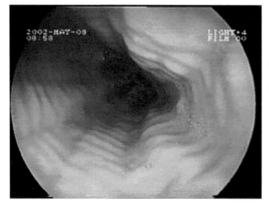

Figure 18.6 Tertiary contraction waves in the esophagus – "feline esophagus."

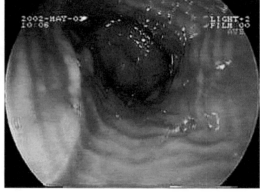

Figure 18.7 Tertiary contraction waves and gastric mucosal prolapse at the distal end of the esophagus.

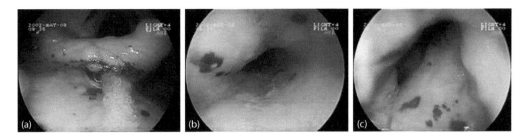

Figure 18.8 Mucosal petechiae in a patient of idiopathic thrombocytopenic purpura (ITP) at (a) the laryngo-pharynx and (b, c) the esophagus.

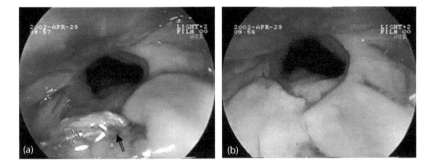

Figure 18.9 (a, b) Esophago-gastric anastomosis. Note the residual suture (arrow).

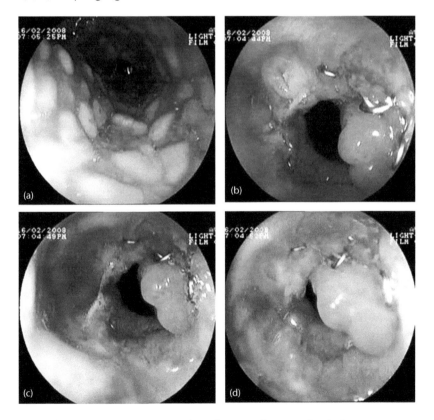

Figure 18.10 Esophago-gastrostomy. (a) Bile reflux esophagitis. (b–d) Tumor recurrence at esophago-gastrostomy site. The patient had undergone proximal gastrectomy for a GE junction tumor. Note the residual sutures at the anastomotic site.

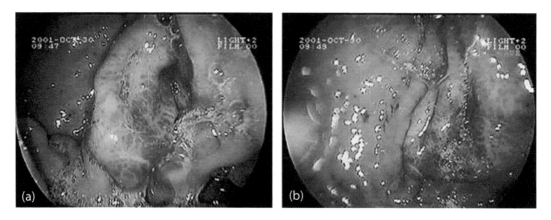

Figure 18.11 Retching gastropathy. (a, b) Congested and ecchymosed gastric mucosa just below the GE junction. This has resulted from repeated prolapse through the LES during the act of retching and vomiting.

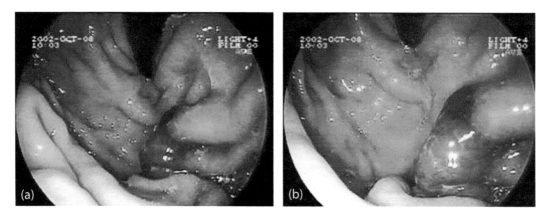

Figure 18.12 Retching gastropathy. (a, b) Focal ecchymosed gastric mucosa just below GE junction.

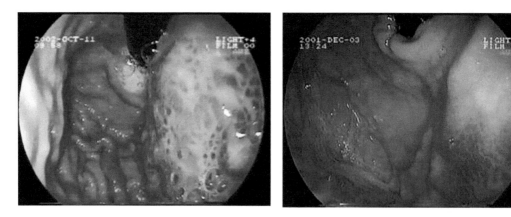

Figure 18.13 Retching gastropathy.

Figure 18.14 Retching gastropathy.

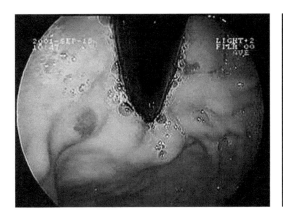

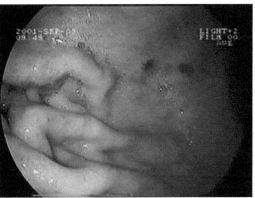

Figure 18.15 Angiodysplasia in the proximal gastric mucosa.

Figure 18.16 Ecchymosis produced by nasogastric tube.

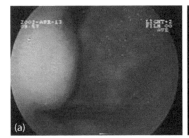
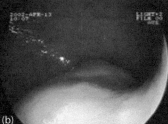
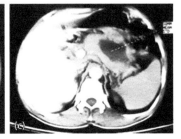

Figure 18.17 (a, b) Pancreatic pseudocyst producing bulge in the proximal stomach. (c) CT scan image of the same patient showing the thick-walled pseudocyst.

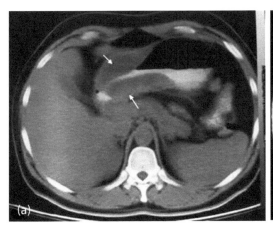
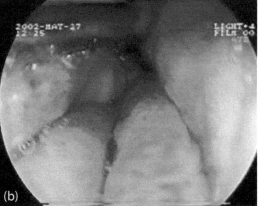

Figure 18.18 (a) CT scan showing gastric intramural pseudocyst. (b) The edematous antral mucosa. Patient, a known case of recurrent pancreatitis presented with gastric outlet obstruction. Previously, he had undergone percutaneous catheter drainage for retrogastric pseudocyst.

American Journal of Gastroenterology 2003; 98: 229

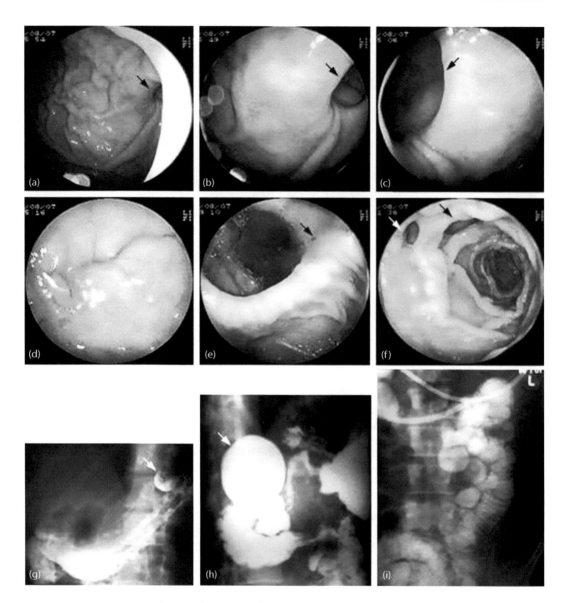

Figure 18.19 (a) Gastric diverticulum in the fundus of the stomach (arrow). (b, c) Close-up view of the same. (d) Dilated blood vessels in the wall of the diverticulum. (e) Giant juxtapapillary diverticulum in the same patient. Note the papillary orifice (arrow) in the wall of the diverticulum. (f) Multiple jejunal diverticuli (arrows) were also noted on enteroscopy. Barium contrast study showing the (g) gastric diverticulum (arrow), (h) juxtapapillary diverticulum (arrow) and (i) jejunal diverticuli. The patient presented with massive lower GI bleeding.

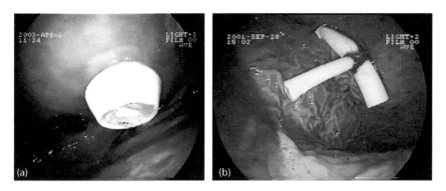

Figure 18.20 **(a)** Percutaneous endoscopic gastrostomy (PEG) tube in the stomach. **(b)** PEG tube, indigenously prepared from Foley's catheter.

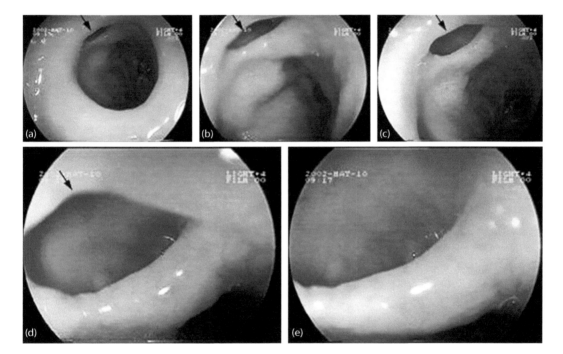

Figure 18.21 **(a–c)** True diverticulum (arrow) in the superior wall of D1. **(d, e)** Close-up view of the same. Note the healthy and normal appearing mucosa inside the diverticulum.

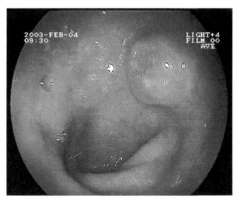

Figure 18.22 Ectopic pancreas in D1. The umbilicated appearance is quite typical.

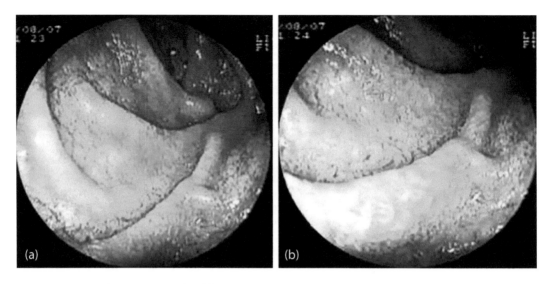

Figure 18.23 (a, b) Brunner's gland hyperplasia imparting a velvety appearance to the duodenal mucosa.

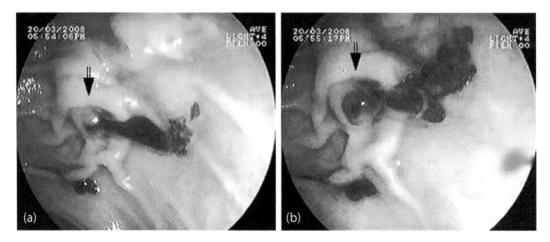

Figure 18.24 Hemobilia. (a, b) Blood emanating from papilla (arrow) in a patient having cholangiocarcinoma.

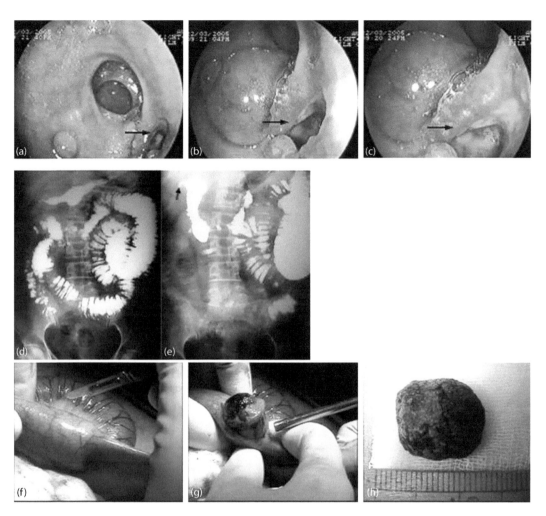

Figure 18.25 Gallstone ileus. **(a–c)** Endoscopic view of D1 showing cholecystoduodenal fistula (arrow). The excavated base of the ulcer is the gallbladder lumen. **(d)** Barium contrast study showing dilated loop of the jejunum. **(e)** Fistula (arrow) delineated on contrast study. **(f)** Impacted stone in the proximal jejunum, **(g)** being delivered by enterotomy. **(h)** The offending stone. The patient, an elderly woman, presented with features of upper small bowel obstruction.

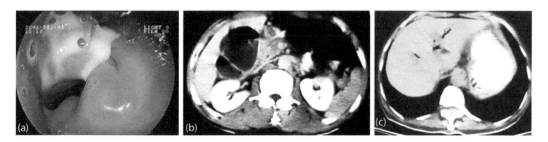

Figure 18.26 **(a)** Cholecystoduodenal fistula. Active pus discharge was noted in D1. **(b)** CT scan showing air inside the distended gallbladder and **(c)** in the intrahepatic biliary radicles. The patient, a known case of gallstone disease, was admitted with acute cholecystitis. Resolution of his symptom coincided with the formation of such fistula, a fact not-so-well described in the literature.

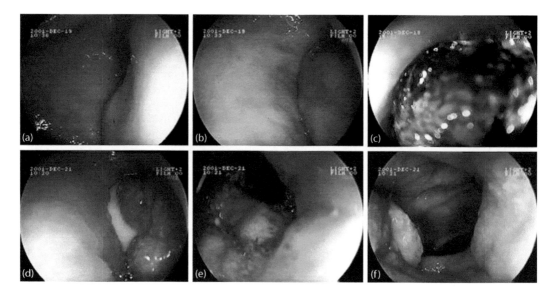

Figure 18.27 Bouvret's syndrome. **(a, b)** An external bulge was noted in the antropyloric region. **(c)** A large size gallstone was found impacted in D1. **(d)** Endoscopy performed 48 h later showed pus discharge from the bulge. **(e)** The gallstone had passed down, the site of impaction showing mucosal irregularity. **(f)** Postbulbar duodenum. The patient presented with gastric outlet obstruction that resolved spontaneously with the passage of the offending stone.

Index

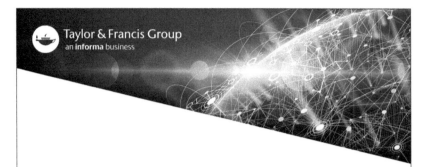